MINDFULNESS-BASED COGNITIVE THERAPY
FOR DEPRESSION

Mindfulness-Based Cognitive Therapy for Depression

A NEW APPROACH TO PREVENTING RELAPSE

Zindel V. Segal

J. Mark G. Williams

John D. Teasdale

Foreword by Jon Kabat-Zinn

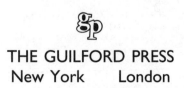

THE GUILFORD PRESS
New York   London

© 2002 The Guilford Press
A Division of Guilford Publications, Inc.
72 Spring Street, New York, NY 10012
www.guilford.com

Printed in the United States of America

This book is printed on acid-free paper.

Last digit is print number: 9   8   7   6   5   4   3

Library of Congress Cataloging-in-Publication Data

Segal, Zindel V., 1956–
    Mindfulness-based cognitive therapy for depression: a new approach
to preventing relapse / Zindel V. Segal, J. Mark G. Williams, John D. Teasdale.
        p. cm.
    Includes bibliographical references and index.
    ISBN 1-57230-706-4 (cloth)
    1. Depression, Mental—Treatment.   2. Cognitive therapy.   I. Williams,
J. Mark G.   II. Teasdale, John D.   III. Title.

RC537 .S44 2002
616.85′270651—dc21

                                                                    2001045051

To Lisa, Ariel, Shira, and Solomon
—Z. V. Segal

To Phyllis, Rob, Jennie, and Annie
—J. M. G. Williams

To Jackie, Joe, and Ben
—J. D. Teasdale

About the Authors

Zindel V. Segal, PhD, holds the Morgan Firestone Chair in Psychotherapy at the University of Toronto. He is Head of Cognitive Behaviour Therapy at the Center for Addiction and Mental Health and Professor of Psychiatry and Psychology at the University of Toronto. He is also the Head of the Psychotherapy Program for the Department of Psychiatry. Dr. Segal is a founding fellow of the Academy of Cognitive Therapy. His publications include *Cognitive Vulnerability to Depression* (with Rick E. Ingram and Jeanne Miranda, 1998).

J. Mark G. Williams, DPhil, is Professor of Clinical Psychology at the University of Wales, Bangor, and since 1997, Director of the University's Institute of Medical and Social Care Research. Widely published, his recent books include *The Psychological Treatment of Depression* (1992), *Cognitive Psychology and Emotional Disorders* (with Fraser Watts, Colin MacLeod, and Andrew Mathews, 1997), and *Cry of Pain: Understanding Suicide and Self-Harm* (1997). He is a founding fellow of the Academy of Cognitive Therapy.

John D. Teasdale, PhD, has researched cognitive models and treatments of depression for more than 20 years. He holds a Special Scientific Appointment at the Medical Research Council's Cognition and Brain Sciences Unit in Cambridge, England. He is a fellow of the British Academy, a fellow of the Academy of Medical Sciences, and a founding fellow of the Academy of Cognitive Therapy. Dr. Teasdale received the American Psychological Association's (Division 12) Distinguished Scientist Award in 1990.

Foreword

Mindfulness-Based Cognitive Therapy for Depression is to my mind a seminal book. It unites for the first time what are commonly thought of as Eastern meditative practices and perspectives (in this case, mindfulness meditation) with Western psychological epistemologies and practices (in this case, cognitive therapy) in a new and seamless synthesis. This novel therapeutic approach was developed in the service of relieving human suffering, especially the emotional suffering that afflicts people experiencing depression. It was also developed in the service of expanding our understanding and treatment of depression. However, the implications of this work go beyond depression and provide potentially useful theoretical and therapeutic windows into a range of affective disorders.

It is also a courageous book in several senses of the word. First, it is courageous because the authors choose to tell it, with great humility, honesty, and passion, as the story of their own learning in encountering and then testing a very different paradigm from that in which they were trained professionally and in which they were recognized as experts. This is an unusual approach for a scientific text, as the authors themselves acknowledge, and one that I think is, in this instance, both admirable and totally appropriate to accomplish their professional purposes given the subject matter. The book is also courageous in the root meaning of the word (*coeur*, in French, for heart).

It ultimately concerns the potential that exists for personal transformation (traditionally expressed as a change in heart as well as mind), both for the authors in their roles as researchers and therapist/instructors, and for their patients. Such transformation is the work of mindfulness itself, brought about by paying attention in highly specific ways to the entire landscape, inner and outer, of one's experiences, including intense emotions. One might call this the path to the embodiment of emotional intelligence.

Mindfulness lies at the core of Buddhist meditative practices, yet its essence is universal. It has to do with refining our capacities for paying attention, for sustained and penetrative awareness, and for emergent insight that is beyond thought but can be articulated through thought. Thus, the practice of mindfulness lends itself beautifully to the kind of synthesis with cognitive therapy reflected in this volume.

Strictly speaking, mindfulness is not a technique or method, although there are many different methods and techniques for its cultivation. Rather, it is more aptly described as a way of being, or a way of seeing, one that involves "coming to one's senses" in every meaning of that phrase. It certainly implies developing and refining a way of becoming more intimate with one's own experience through systematic self-observation. This includes intentionally suspending the impulse to characterize, evaluate, and judge what one is experiencing. Doing so affords multiple opportunities to move beyond the well-worn grooves of our highly conditioned and largely habitual and unexamined thought processes and emotional reactivity.

Because the field of experience to which intentional mindfulness can be brought is so broad (including, inwardly, sensations, perceptions, impulses, emotions, thoughts, and the process of thinking itself; and outwardly, speech, actions, and relationships), it has huge potential for helping those who suffer from emotional difficulties. It was the convergence of, on the one hand, the latest theories of how cognitive therapies have their effects, and, on the other, the mindfulness approach—of seeing thoughts as thoughts, as events in the field of awareness, independent of their content and their emotional "charge," without trying to change them, replace them with other thoughts, or "fix" anything, but rather observe them with a degree of equanimity—that encouraged the authors to seek to build a bridge between these two perspectives. This book reports what happened when they began to build that bridge; how they observed that the attentional practices of mindfulness meditation and the intentions behind them seemed to facilitate a deepening of self-knowledge and self-acceptance in their patients. These transformations in view and understanding in turn appeared to have profound short- and long-term effects on health and well-being, as suggested by the clinical and research findings reported here. In the end, the authors found it possible to apply their firsthand experience and understanding from the laboratory of their own meditation practice, coupled with their profound expertise in cognitive therapy and cognitive science, to the problem of depression in creative ways that have given rise to a new therapeutic approach, namely, mindfulness-based cognitive therapy.

The adaptation of the more generic mindfulness-based stress reduction approach to a specific clinical disorder capitalizes on the potential value of mindfulness meditation as a practice that can speak to the deep soul needs of individuals. It appears to be accessible to and enthusiastically adopted by a wide range of people. Practitioners often report that they benefit from and actually enjoy the cultivation of greater awareness and self-knowledge, painful as it sometimes can be, because of its authenticity, its grounding in felt experience embraced in nonjudging awareness. Practitioners report finding new degrees of freedom associated with the ongoing cultivation of mindfulness in dealing skillfully with both the larger world and the terrain of their own interiority.

It is my sincere hope that this book will introduce mindfulness to both clinicians and researchers in the cognitive therapy community in ways that will spark interest and enthusiasm and will benefit people suffering from depression. I hope that it will also introduce those primarily interested in mindfulness meditation to recent developments in understanding the psychological processes that underlie recurrent depressive disorders, for the usefulness of a well-built bridge is that it can take traffic in both directions. The remarkable synthesis that this book represents holds the promise not only of developing our theories of how cognition and emotion interact, but also of furthering our understanding of the deep inner capacities of human beings for healing and for living lives of greater wisdom, balance, and happiness.

JON KABAT-ZINN, PhD
Center for Mindfulness in Medicine,
Health Care, and Society
University of Massachusetts Medical School

Acknowledgments

It is a pleasure to acknowledge, with gratitude, all those who, at different times and in different ways, have supported the development and evaluation of mindfulness-based cognitive therapy (MBCT) and the writing of this book. Here, we name some persons, but our thanks extend also to many whom we do not name. In Toronto, we thank Mark Lau, Michael Gemar, Susan Williams, and Neil Rector. In Bangor, we thank Judith Soulsby, Sarah Silverton, Rebecca Crane, Sheila Jenkins, Keith Fearns, and Isabel Hargreaves. In Cambridge, we thank Surbala Morgan, Valerie Ridgeway, Sally Cox, and Helen Ma. Our external readers, Anne Simons, Andy MacLeod, Jackie Teasdale, Ben Teasdale, and Carol Garson, provided invaluable feedback on an early draft of the book and helped us to appreciate more clearly what was needed for the book's final assembly.

This book is not just an account of how we developed a treatment to prevent depressive relapse. It also chronicles our own stepwise accommodation to a very different paradigm for working with depression and its aftermath. In both areas, we were extraordinarily fortunate to have the steadfast guidance, support, and wisdom of Jon Kabat-Zinn and the staff of the Center for Mindfulness in Medicine, Health Care, and Society, especially Saki Santorelli, Ferris Urbanowski, and Elana Rosenbaum. We know that we have included a great deal of material from the Stress Reduction Clinic at the University of Massachusetts (UMass) and from Jon Kabat-Zinn's *Full Catastrophe Living*, and we remain very grateful to the clinic staff for their openness to our using their material. Without their guidance, this project, in the form that it developed, would, quite simply, not have been possible.

We are also aware of how much our own thinking, as well as our teaching, has been influenced by other members of the mindfulness community, by their books and tapes, and by workshops we attended and talks we heard. Christina Feldman had a powerful influence on both what we taught and the style in which we taught, as did other insight meditation teachers, especially Sharon Salzberg, Joseph Goldstein, Jack Kornfield, and Larry Rosenberg, whose written and spoken words sharpened our understanding of the heart of mindfulness practice. Wherever we can trace a specific source for the way these teachers have influenced how we teach MBCT, we have acknowledged it, but we suspect that many of these influences may have become incorporated implicitly into our own approach, and we apologize if there is material we have failed to acknowledge.

This work was initially supported by the John D. and Catherine T. MacArthur Foundation Research Network on the Psychobiology of Depression and Other Affective Disorders, chaired by David J. Kupfer. It was also funded by Grant No. RA 013 from the Wales Office of Research and Development for Health and Social Care, and by Grant No. MH53457 from the National Institute of Mental Health. Our personal support came from the Center for Addiction and Mental Health, the University of Wales, and the Medical Research Council of the United Kingdom.

We would also like to thank Barbara Watkins, our editor at The Guilford Press, who worked steadfastly to help us see how, in a manuscript written for multiple audiences, we could find a way to address them in a single voice.

Finally, our thanks and heartfelt appreciation go out to the courageous patients who took part in the MBCT groups. We are grateful to them for allowing us to reflect their experiences in this book. Working with them was, for us, an inspiration and an education. We are delighted that it was also of benefit to many of them.

Contents

Part III
EVALUATION AND DISSEMINATION

MINDFULNESS-BASED COGNITIVE THERAPY FOR DEPRESSION

PART I

&

The Challenge
of Depression

Introduction

Most books start with a preface. The trouble is that many people don't read prefaces, which is a pity. In the preface, the authors are normally more relaxed. They tell you how they came to write the book—the meetings, the problems, and how such problems were overcome. Warm acknowledgments to funding agencies and colleagues exist side by side with warmer acknowledgments to partners and children. Then comes Chapter 1, often accompanied by a distinct change in temperature that can last until the end of the book. Here is a different climate: the academic literature, the intricate theory, the complexities of therapy. In a preface, we might have been allowed to make all sorts of personal statements, and express all sorts of doubts. But once started, the book allows no such indulgence; it should be hermetically sealed from such observations.

Each of the authors of this book has written such texts, so we understand what such books can and cannot do. We do not mean to condemn our own past efforts. But we have resolved that this will be a different sort of book. We would like it to say how we came to develop an approach to the treatment of depression that was new to each of us. More than that, the approach was born out of our attempts to discover a way to tackle one of the biggest problems about depression: its tendency to recur once a person has suffered it once. This book tells how we came to believe that this approach to depression was worth pursuing. Of course, part of the story is about how we were influenced by the academic literature and our own research findings; how we attempted (again and again) to get a better theoretical understanding of recurrent depression; and how we chose to implement these understandings in what has come to be known as mindfulness-based cognitive therapy (MBCT). We also describe MBCT in some detail. So, no preface; just a story. As with all stories, we begin at the beginning (or one of them), back in the summer of 1989.

How we started to work together on this project is briefly and easily told. Mark Williams and John Teasdale both worked at the Medical Research Council's Applied Psychology Unit in Cambridge, England, and Zindel Segal visited them in 1989, en route to the World Congress of Cognitive Therapy, which was meeting in Oxford that year. The three of us had worked on psychological models and treatment of depression. We were each to present papers at the Congress: Mark Williams on the subject of chronic and recurrent depression, Zindel Segal on the interaction of life stress and relapse, and John Teasdale on a new model of how cognition and emotion might interrelate.

The discussion at that pre-Congress meeting in Cambridge was about the puzzles that recent research on cognition and emotion was throwing up and whether advances in this area could be applied to explain how negative thinking and feelings combine in depression with such debilitating results. Perhaps because we had each pursued different leads in investigating a common problem, namely, how depression alters people's thinking, there was a good deal to share. At that time, both Mark Williams and Zindel Segal were studying how depression changes a person's view of him- or herself. Mark Williams was studying the different types of personal memories that accompany depression, whereas Zindel Segal was measuring depressed patients' self-images by examining the time they took to respond to negative and positive information about themselves. John Teasdale was moving away from measures that rely on a single level of meaning. Instead, he was exploring the possibility that shifts at a more holistic level of meaning, involving whole mind states, might be responsible for the particular emotional changes found in depression. This work eventually developed into a comprehensive model of cognition and emotion relationships known as *interacting cognitive subsystems*.[1]

It is interesting that our conversations were largely about the mechanisms that lie behind the changes in thinking and feeling that accompany depression. We were not focusing our attention on the treatment of depression, because by the late 1980s there were already a number of psychological treatments whose effects were on par with those found for antidepressant medication. Further research on how to help people with current depression seemed unlikely, at that time, to add much to the field.

Instead, we focused our interest on how we could better predict which persons were most likely to become depressed again once they had recovered from an episode of depression. The academic literature was uncertain. Some early studies seemed to suggest that if people continued to hold certain attitudes about themselves or the world after recovery, then they would be the ones most likely to become depressed again. Examples include the beliefs "If I do not do as well as other people, it means I am an inferior human being" or "My value as a person depends greatly on what others think of me." Such beliefs or assumptions were thought to make depression more likely, largely because they link a person's self-esteem with events that, large or small, are often outside his or her control. A questionnaire called the Dysfunctional Attitude Scale had been developed to measure the degree to which people held such beliefs.

Increasingly, researchers were skeptical of the role of these attitudes in relapse. They pointed out that patients who still held these sorts of beliefs at the end of treatment may not have fully recovered, so it was no wonder that they were more likely to relapse. Indeed, several other studies showed that patients who had truly recovered, so that their depressed mood had returned to the average level of the general population, showed no evidence of this type of thinking style. Their attitude scores were normal despite the fact that these people, we knew, were very likely to become depressed again. In what way could these people be shown to be vulnerable? We continued to debate this question at the time, and we have more to say about it later. In any case, the Oxford Congress came and went, and, promising to keep in touch, we returned to our own academic homes.

Two years later, in 1991, there arose the opportunity to come together again to focus on the same issues. David Kupfer, who headed the Psychobiology of Depression Research Network of the John D. and Catherine T. MacArthur Foundation, had asked Zindel Segal to develop a "maintenance" version of cognitive therapy for use with depressed patients once they had recovered from their acute episode. Maintenance therapy offered a way to continue treating recovered but at-risk individuals. It was offered less frequently than regular therapy and supported formerly depressed patients' use of skills to identify and address problems that, if ignored, could bring on depression. David Kupfer and Ellen Frank had just published a seminal study on maintenance interpersonal therapy. Could a maintenance version of cognitive therapy be similarly developed? Zindel, who was now Head of the Cognitive Behaviour Therapy Unit at the Clarke Institute of Psychiatry, contacted Mark Williams (who had moved from Cambridge to the Chair of Clinical Psychology at the University of Wales at Bangor) and John Teasdale to discuss the possibility of working together on such a project. Our first meeting was in Toronto, in April 1992. The notes from that meeting outline what such a maintenance cognitive therapy treatment would look like. It bears no resemblance to the approach we describe in this book. In the coming years, we would radically depart from the version of cognitive therapy in which each of us had been trained.

As Part I of this book explains, we first stepped away by adding an attentional training component to our cognitive therapy intervention and then discarded the "therapy" framework to work more fully within a mindfulness approach that emphasized holding thoughts and feelings in awareness rather than trying to change them. How we finally moved towards an integration of core cognitive therapy principles with sustained mindfulness practice is the longer story we now endeavor to tell.

We begin by giving some background on depression itself. There was no doubt in our minds from the outset that depression posed one of the most pressing problems in the field of mental health. What did the situation look like in the late 1980s, and what new perspectives were emerging? We shall see that views of depression were changing, from depression as a single-episode problem, to depression as a chronic, recurrent disorder. Health planners were beginning to wake up to the fact that depression was poised to be one of the major "diseases" of the 21st century, demanding new answers.

CHAPTER I

8

Depression

THE SCOPE OF THE PROBLEM

Depression in its broadest sense is a disorder of mood. In its common usage the term suggests that one is "feeling down" or "blue," yet this characterization misses the essential "syndromal" nature of the clinical disorder, that is, it consists of a combination of elements rather than a single feature. Clinical depression (sometimes also called "major depression") is a state in which persistent depressed mood or loss of interest occurs together with other reliable physical and mental signs, such as difficulties sleeping, poor appetite, impaired concentration, and feelings of hopelessness and worthlessness. A diagnosis of depression is only given when a number of these elements are present at the same time, for at least 2 weeks, and are shown to interfere with a person's ability to perform his or her day-to-day activities.

When we consider how many people suffer from depression, the figures are staggering. Based on data from both hospital and community studies, such mood disorders are among the most prevalent psychiatric conditions, a finding that is remarkably consistent all over the world. Recent epidemiological data from roughly 14,000 patients surveyed across six European countries found that 17% of the population report some experience with depression in the past 6 months. When looked at more closely, major depression accounted for 6.9%, with minor depression accounting for 1.8%.[2] The remaining 8.3% of subjects complained of experiencing depressive symptoms but did not view them as interfering greatly with either their work or social functioning. These numbers are closely comparable to rates reported in both Canadian[3] and U.S. samples.[4] At these levels, family physicians can expect to see at least one person with a significant depression during each day of clinical practice. When people are asked about their experiences with depression over longer periods of time, the figures are, of course, higher. At any one time, 10% of the U.S. population have experienced clinical depression in the past year[5] and between 20–25% of women and 7–12% of men will suffer a clinical depression during their lifetime.[6]

Those who have been depressed know that there is no single face to the disorder, no single feature that tells the whole story. Some consequences of having depression are easier to recognize by the sufferer, including low mood and lack of concentration. Others may be harder to recognize because their main effects reduce the patient's ability to interact with loved ones and other family members, for example, lack of energy, preoccupation with negative themes and ideas. One of the most obvious tolls that depression exacts is increased risk for suicide. Suicide risk increases with each new episode, and there is a 15% chance that patients suffering from recurrent depression severe enough to require hospitalization will eventually die by suicide.[7] Depression is also rarely observed on its own. The most likely additional problem is anxiety.[8] The chances of a person with depression, for example, also suffering from panic disorder are 19 times greater than the odds of someone without depression experiencing panic.[9,10] Increased odds are also reported for simple phobia (nine times greater) and obsessive–compulsive disorder (11 times greater).

One of the most surprising and disturbing aspects to emerge from community-based surveys of depression and other mental illnesses is the low rate of use of mental health services. There is a strange irony here. People with the most prevalent mental disorder are among the least likely to seek treatment. The number of depressed persons who do not seek mental health services is greater than the number who are treated. People who are depressed, like others with mental health problems, are reluctant to seek treatment: Only 12% actually see a specialist for their problem.[5] The failure to obtain care, especially in the case of depression for which effective treatments exist, has developed into an important public health issue. One response to this has been publicity to educate the public about the symptoms of depression and available treatment options. Depression screening days are now common in many hospitals and have helped to reduce the stigma associated with this disorder by portraying it as a legitimate medical/psychological condition with well-documented clinical features.

Another change in our understanding of depression that has occurred over the past 10 years has been to appreciate the degree of disability associated with the disorder. In addition to the emotional pain and anguish suffered by those who are depressed, recent evidence suggests that the level of functional impairment is comparable to that found in major medical illnesses, including cancer and coronary artery disease. The work of Kenneth Wells and his colleagues has gone far in revealing many of the hidden costs and the nature of the social burden due to depression. For example, when we measure disability in terms of "days spent in bed," many people would be surprised to find that depressed patients spent more time in bed (1.4 days per month) than patients with lung disease (1.2 days per month), diabetes (1.15 days per month) or arthritis (0.75 days per month). Only patients with heart disease spent more time in bed (2.1 days per month).[11] As one might assume, the ripple effect of "bed days" on productivity at work is considerable. Workers suffering from depression have five times more work-loss days than do their healthy counterparts,[12] and depression is one of the most common causes of extended work absence in white-collar employees.[13]

The impact of these findings, as they entered the literature in the late 1980s and early 1990s, was that many people changed their views on the magnitude of the problem of depression. A recent World Health Organization projection for the year 2020 estimates that, of all diseases, depression will impose the second-largest burden of ill health worldwide.[10] At the time we came together to consider the best treatment approach to depression, it was fast becoming the major challenge within the field of mental health.

EARLY OPTIMISM ABOUT THE TREATMENT OF DEPRESSION

If depression was the problem, where was the answer likely to be found? The truth was that by the end of the 1980s, there were a number of ways to combat depression. Antidepressant drugs, first discovered and used in the 1950s, had been refined to the point that a number of them had amassed decisive evidence for their efficacy. Most of these drugs targeted brain neurotransmitter function (the chemical messengers that allow neural impulses to cross from one nerve fiber to another at their junctions, or synapses). They worked by increasing the efficiency of the connections between brain cells and making greater quantities of neurotransmitters, such as norepinephrine or serotonin, available at the synapse.[14] Although how exactly this occurs remains in doubt, there is evidence to suggest that some drugs block the reuptake of neurotransmitters by other cells, whereas others actually stimulate nerve cells to release more neurotransmitter. By the end of the 1980s antidepressants had become, and still remain, the frontline treatment for clinical depression.[15]

Psychological treatments of depression were also starting to come into their own. There were at least four broad approaches to the problem, all of which were structured and time-limited. Each had some degree of empirical support by the mid-1980s. Behavioral approaches emphasized the need to increase depressed persons' participation in reinforcing or pleasure-giving activities,[16] while social skills training corrected behavioral deficits that increased depressed persons' social isolation and rejection.[17] Cognitive therapy[18] brought together a number of behavioral and cognitive techniques, with the joint aim of changing the way a person's thoughts, images, and interpretation of events contribute to the onset and maintenance of the emotional and behavioral disturbances associated with depression. Finally, interpersonal therapy[19] stressed that learning to resolve interpersonal disputes and changing roles would alleviate depression. There were also hybrid interventions such as Rehm's self-control therapy.[20] This group treatment combined features of the behavioral and cognitive approaches to teach depressed persons how to evaluate, monitor, and reward themselves in light of realistic rather than perfectionistic standards. Cognitive and interpersonal therapies came to be seen as the gold standards in psychological treatment, largely because the support for these interventions reflected three important features: The therapies were tested in multiple studies conducted in different centers; they used clinical patients who met standard diagnostic criteria for depression; and when evaluated against antidepressant medication, their efficacy was judged to be equivalent.[21]

With all these treatments for depression available, surely the problem had been solved. Unfortunately, as treatments for current depression demonstrated their efficacy, research showed that a major contributor to prevalence rates across the world was the *return* of new episodes of depression in people who had already experienced one episode. The scope of the problem had changed.

DEPRESSION AS A CHRONIC, RELAPSING CONDITION

Why had this aspect of depression not been noticed before? Because, to come to this conclusion, one needs studies in which patients who have recovered from the disorder are followed and evaluated at regular intervals. Only with this type of information can there be a complete understanding of how depression waxes and wanes over the lifecycle, and how its natural course develops. Such studies allow us to calculate the likelihood of spontaneous remission (in which a person gets better without treatment) and to evaluate the relative costs of using treatments that carry significant risks or side effects against the costs of leaving depression untreated. There was little in the way of hard data on these issues until the mid 1980s. One barrier to collecting this type of information is that identifying new cases of depression and just passively observing the effects of the disorder is not ethically feasible. It is unethical not to offer treatment for depression. This means that there are no untreated depressed patients who could be followed for years. More patients, however, were receiving and responding to treatment. Instead of simply studying the way depression changed in response to treatment, newer studies identified patients once they were no longer depressed, then followed them over 1- to 2-year intervals.

One of the first such studies was conducted by Martin Keller and colleagues in 1983.[22] His group followed 141 patients diagnosed with major depressive disorder for 13 months and reported that 43 (33%) had relapsed after having been well for at least 8 weeks. Clearly, patients in recovery faced a major challenge in maintaining their health and the gains of treatment. More recent estimates suggest that at least 50% of patients who recover from an initial episode of depression will have at least one subsequent depressive episode,[23] and those patients with a history of two or more past episodes will have a 70–80% likelihood of recurrence in their lives.[6] Up to this point, mental health professionals had distinguished "acute" conditions (short-term) from "chronic" conditions (long-term; lasting over 2 years), noting that some depressions might *appear* acute, but that many depressed people who had recovered remained "chronic" in the sense of increased, long-term vulnerability. In a widely quoted review, Judd concluded that "unipolar depression is a chronic, lifelong illness, the risk for repeated episodes exceeds 80%, patients will experience an average of 4 lifetime major depressive episodes of 20 weeks' duration each" (p. 990).[24] Findings such as these have helped to shape the current consensus that relapse and recurrence following successful treatment of depression are common, debilitating outcomes.

From the perspective of the early part of the 21st century, it is easy to forget that this emphasis on recurrence was quite new at the time. Up to the late 1960s and early 1970s, the focus had been on developing more effective treatments for acute depression. Relatively little attention was paid to a patient's ongoing risk. Keller's work signaled the need to take into account the risk of relapse that remained during recovery, when making decisions about the type of treatment to offer.

Keller's data suggested a large difference in prognosis between patients with no past history of depression and those with at least three previous depressive episodes. These two groups relapsed at significantly different rates—22% for "first timers" versus 67% for patients with a past history of three or more episodes. Patients recovering from their first episode of depression were shown to be at a critical juncture in the development of the course of their disorder. They "have a substantial probability of prompt relapse, and should they relapse, they have approximately a 20% chance of remaining chronically depressed" (p. 3303).[22] As later data from a 5-year follow-up of patients with chronic and nonchronic affective disorder suggested,[25] those who relapse very soon after recovery are the ones whose depression becomes a long-lasting condition.

Distinguishing among patients on the basis of the number of past episodes continues to be one of the most reliable predictors of future depression, bearing out Keller's earlier observations. While the threshold in Keller's study was set at three past episodes, now the more common cutoff is two episodes. It is important to note that the principle of separating these two groups on the basis of their risk for relapse is still endorsed. In fact, the *Diagnostic and Statistical Manual of Mental Disorders* of the American Psychiatric Association[26] qualifies the diagnosis of major depressive disorder with the term "recurrent" for those patients with a history of at least two depressive episodes. More recently, the work of Michael Thase[27] has helped to map the biological characteristics of this group of patients, by demonstrating that they have more marked disturbances in their sleep patterns; overactivity in the neuroendocrine system responsible for producing the stress hormone, cortisol; more "endogenous" symptoms of depression (such as early morning wakening and worse mood in the mornings); and depression that often tends not to vary with changing circumstances.

HOW COULD DEPRESSIVE RELAPSE AND RECURRENCE BE PREVENTED?

With a clearer view of the burdens that depression imposes on its sufferers came a corresponding urgency to develop treatments that might help. Because major depression was now seen to be a recurrent disorder, it seemed imperative to look at ways of expanding the types of care offered to patients. The evidence seemed to suggest that if one relied on medication, there was a need for a longer-term approach.

Although the conclusion was not wholly welcome to those uncomfortable with long-term administration of medication, the evidence implied that a clinician should continue to prescribe antidepressants to depressed patients after they had recovered from the episode for which they sought help in the first place. What sort of study could be used to test the necessity of such continuation treatment?

The answer is a study in which all patients receive the same medication until they have recovered, and are then randomly allocated either to a condition in which the active drug is swapped for a placebo (an inert pill) or one in which they continue to receive the active drug. (Patients agree beforehand to participate in such a study but do not know the group to which they are assigned). That is what Glen and his colleagues did in a seminal study in the early 1980s. All patients were allocated to receive drug or placebo once they had got better on the active drug. The results were clear: Some 50% of the patients who were switched to the placebo became depressed again, compared to only 20% of the patients treated with active medication.[28]

One feature of this result was particularly important. Glen et al. found that depression came back much more quickly than would be expected if it were a new episode. This suggested that patients were not experiencing a new episode (a "recurrence") but, rather, the worsening of a previously controlled episode that had not yet run its course (a "relapse"). The more general implication of this result was that, although persons suffering an episode of depression might feel better after taking antidepressant medication, if they stopped the medication before the episode had run its course, they risked rapid relapse.

By the late 1980s, many clinicians endorsed the view that it was best to prevent future episodes of depression by prescribing antidepressant medication prophylactically (i.e., to prevent the occurrence of a future episode, and not just to treat the existing episode). Clinicians started to distinguish between acute, continuation, and maintenance use of antidepressant medication to refer to treatment at the different stages of the depression. So prescribing antidepressants with the aim of relieving current symptoms during an episode, was called acute treatment. Prescribing antidepressants for 6 months beyond the period of recovery from the episode of depression was called continuation treatment, and when extended for as long as 3 to 5 years following recovery, it was referred to as maintenance treatment. The American Psychiatric Association's current practice guidelines for depression are based on this framework.[29,30]

But note a very important assumption behind these guidelines: that antidepressant drugs do not provide a long-term cure. Their effects do not outlast their use. To put it another way, antidepressants have their effects by suppressing symptoms; they do not target the supposed causes of the episode itself.[31,32] Nevertheless, given that the risk for early recurrence increases with each episode experienced, and that the interval between recurrences tends to shorten over time,[33] it remained important to prevent the return of symptoms in any way possible. For many, the message of this and similar, later studies was clear: To prevent future depression, continue the same treatments that worked in alleviating the acute episode of depression.

PSYCHOTHERAPY AS A MAINTENANCE TREATMENT

The gains achieved through extending pharmacological treatment of depression beyond initial recovery were, by the late 1980s, well documented and extremely important. Yet effective alternatives to the continued use of antidepressant medication in the recovery phase were still required. At any given time, there is a considerable number of people for whom such long-term drug treatment is not suitable. For example, pregnant women are discouraged from taking such medication, as are those undergoing major surgery. Others cannot tolerate the side effects of antidepressants, and still others decline to take the medication. In a study of 155 depressed outpatients, 28% stopped taking antidepressants during the first month of treatment, and 44% had stopped taking their medication by the third month.[34] In general, the proportion of patients who do not take the prescribed antidepressant medication is estimated in the 30–40% range.[35] A

recent online survey of 1,400 patients in the United States, conducted by the National Depressive and Manic–Depressive Association, found that only one-third of patients receiving maintenance
antidepressant therapy were satisfied with the quality of their treatment.[36]

Could psychotherapy help? After all, there was evidence that
negative life events often precede the return of episodes of depression. Such events often involve losses, arguments, rejections, and disappointments. Surely, then, psychotherapy could play an important
role in helping patients manage the interpersonal consequences of
these events, thus reducing the risk of recurrence. This was the rationale behind the groundbreaking study of maintenance interpersonal
psychotherapy conducted by Ellen Frank and her colleagues.[37]

What was new about this study was that patients were first
treated for their episode of depression with a combination of interpersonal therapy and the antidepressant, imipramine, and then continued to receive therapy for 3 years, even though they had already
recovered. For patients, the experimental part of the study started
once they had recovered from their episode of depression. One hundred twenty-eight patients who had responded to treatment were
then assigned to one of five groups for a 3-year period: maintenance
alone, maintenance interpersonal therapy and placebo, imipramine
alone, imipramine and maintenance interpersonal therapy, or placebo alone.

The effectiveness of maintenance psychotherapy over the follow-
up period can be gauged by comparing patients who received only
placebo with those who received only monthly maintenance interpersonal therapy. Statistical analysis of relapse and recurrence uses
"survival analysis," a technique derived from studies of treatment for
people with terminal illness. In these cases, the investigator is interested in whether a treatment can prolong life. Rather ominously, psychologists and psychiatrists now use the same term for how long a
person stays well before he or she becomes depressed again. Results
from Ellen Frank's study showed that maintenance interpersonal
therapy significantly extended such "survival time." For patients who
received maintenance interpersonal therapy, the average survival

time until the next episode was greater than 1 year. By contrast, patients receiving only placebo during the maintenance phase had a depression-free period of only 21 weeks.

How much of this improvement was due to the interpersonal therapy itself? When audiotapes of the therapy sessions were rated to see how well the therapists applied the principles outlined in the interpersonal therapy manual, the answer seemed clear. Patients whose sessions were rated as containing more elements of interpersonal therapy, or a higher "dosage" of the treatment, did not have another episode for, on average, 2 years. By contrast, patients whose treatment was less specifically interpersonal therapy—with fewer interpersonal therapy elements detected in rated sessions—became depressed again, on average, 5 months later.[38]

These findings spoke directly to central concerns in the field. First, they demonstrated that psychotherapy, like antidepressant medication, could reduce the chances that depression would return. Patients receiving medication actually survived longer than those receiving only maintenance interpersonal therapy. However, patients on maintenance interpersonal therapy still did much better than patients receiving only placebo. Second, it was exciting that here was a study showing a link between specific skills taught to patients and the prevention of depressive relapse/recurrence. The more elements of interpersonal therapy that had been taught, the longer patients were able to stay well. In summary, these findings opened the door to using psychotherapy as a preventive measure and challenged the field to develop theoretical models to clarify which skills depressed patients ought to be taught to prevent relapse.

The finding that interpersonal therapy could be used in a maintenance format to keep people well was very important, and it was not long before clinicians started to wonder if other forms of psychotherapy might also be used in this way. The problem was that, at the time, many psychotherapy researchers had put their energies into developing better and more effective treatments for acute depression, and had not considered developing "maintenance" versions of their therapies. If this field was to progress, others would need to do what Ellen Frank and her colleagues had done, and begin to examine how best to offer psychological treatments to keep people well once they had recovered.

The possibility of developing a maintenance version of cognitive therapy to parallel the maintenance version of interpersonal therapy provoked the interest of members of the John D. and Catherine T. MacArthur Foundation's recently formed Psychobiology of Depression and Affective Disorders Research Network. The network director, David Kupfer, invited Zindel Segal to explore how to produce such a maintenance treatment. David Kupfer was also to play an important role later in the development of our ideas, when he allowed us to stray from our initial brief and to follow our growing feeling that such a maintenance form of cognitive therapy was too narrow an approach. But we are running ahead of our story. We were asked to develop a maintenance version of cognitive therapy, and that is where we started.

CHAPTER 2

⁂

Cognition, Mood, and the Nature of Depressive Relapse

DEVELOPING A MAINTENANCE VERSION OF COGNITIVE THERAPY

In April 1992, the three of us met as a group to discuss the possibilities of developing a maintenance version of cognitive therapy. We were optimistic about being able to adapt current cognitive therapy for depression in a way that could be applied to patients in recovery. We believed that such a treatment would draw on skills patients had learned during the acute phase of treatment. In order to understand why this therapy was a good place to start, it may be helpful to provide a brief background.

Cognitive therapy was pioneered by Aaron T. Beck in the 1960s and 1970s as a structured, time-limited approach to depression. Beck had noticed how often the themes of loss, failure, worthlessness, and rejection were featured in the thinking of his depressed patients. Up until this time, most clinicians had assumed that this negative thinking was merely a surface feature of depression, caused by an underlying biological disturbance or psychodynamic conflict. According to these prevailing views, if the underlying problem were treated, then the thoughts would get better.

Beck realized that the causal sequence could work equally well the other way around. Negative thinking could itself *cause* depression. In addition, even if such thinking had not been the first cause of an episode, it could certainly maintain the episode once it had started. For example, if a person believes 100% that "I've got no friends" or "Nobody likes or respects me," then he or she will be less likely to phone a friend for support or to accept invitations, and as a result will become more isolated. This sequence of events will make the person's recovery from low mood even more difficult. Thoughts and feelings could interact with each other in a damaging, vicious spiral.

Beck's therapy took these thoughts seriously. He encouraged his patients to "catch" whatever thought was going through their minds when their mood shifted. They would write the thoughts down and bring them to therapy sessions, where they could be evaluated in the light of evidence for and against them. Homework was scheduled, during which patients would gather more evidence and gradually extend their activities to restore a sense of mastery and pleasure in their daily lives. Difficult situations for patients were cognitively rehearsed during the therapy session, and alternative options to tackling them generated and discussed. Patients were taught to be vigilant for long-term beliefs, attitudes, and assumptions they might hold, and to look out for situations where these might trigger depressed mood.

It is interesting now to reflect on why cognitive therapy became so successful. Partly it was because Beck used evidence from both the clinic and the experimental laboratory to substantiate his ideas, drawing in a wide range of clinicians and academics. He also incorporated many behavioral techniques that shared features with the widely used behavior therapies for anxiety-based problems. But success was equally due to Beck's insistence on carefully assessing both processes and outcomes with valid and reliable measures, on applying the therapy to an important clinical problem that structured psychotherapies had neglected, and on evaluating the treatment against the standard existing treatment (antidepressant medication). Any one of these factors might have made cognitive therapy prominent in the field, but with all of them combined, the case for using this approach with depressed patients was overwhelming, and by the time we were meeting, cognitive therapy had become a (if not *the*) major psychotherapeutic alternative to medication.

If we were to plan a maintenance form of cognitive therapy, it would clearly make most sense for patients to use many of the same techniques to prevent future depression: activity scheduling, rating mastery and pleasure, thought monitoring and challenging, cognitive rehearsal, generating alternative options, and noticing and dealing with dysfunctional attitudes. A maintenance treatment might consist of monthly meetings in which these skills were renewed, deepened, and practiced. It would also make sense for the therapy to inform and train patients to notice early indicators of relapse or recurrence.

At this point, the question of what such a manual for maintenance cognitive therapy would contain seemed relatively uncontroversial. We noticed that colleagues of ours, such as Robin Jarrett, had adopted a similar strategy in developing prophylactic interventions for depression (eventually published in 1998).[39] There seemed to be an emerging consensus that the cognitive therapy approach to prevention of depressive relapse/recurrence should primarily depend on continuing to use those cognitive techniques that were helpful in treating the acute episode.

However, it was not long before our discussions led us to ask whether we should consider alternative approaches. First, we had become aware of the sheer enormity of the problem of depression (see Chapter 1), compared with the scarce resources of psychotherapy. The number of trained cognitive therapists was clearly not going to meet the demand, so to ask such therapists to add maintenance therapy to their already busy caseloads was only likely to prevent them from seeing newly referred patients. There needed to be a more cost-efficient solution than to continue to rely on one-to-one psychotherapy. The second problem with believing that maintenance cognitive therapy would be the answer to relapse was that, by 1992, it was becoming clear that treating acute depression with "standard" cognitive therapy already prevented relapse in many patients.

THE LONG-LASTING EFFECTS
OF COGNITIVE THERAPY

Up to that point, four studies had compared cognitive therapy with antidepressants for the treatment of acute depression, and examined how patients fared over the next 12 to 24 months after initial recovery.[40-43] Patients whose medication was discontinued upon their recovery had, as expected, fairly high rates of relapse/recurrence (varying between 50 and 78%), as shown in Figure 2.1.

However, Figure 2.1 also shows that the proportion of patients who relapsed or needed further treatment was substantially reduced if cognitive therapy alone was used to treat the depression. In this case, rates of recurrence were reduced to 20–36%. These studies, conducted both in the United States and in the United Kingdom,

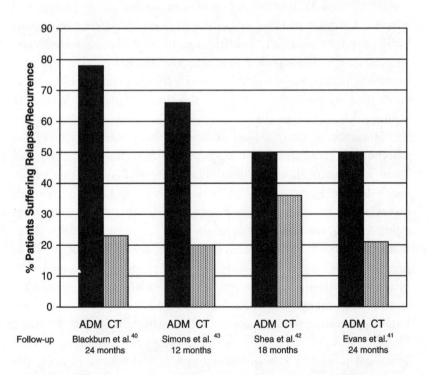

FIGURE 2.1. Comparison of relapse rates for depressed patients receiving either cognitive therapy (CT) or antidepressant medication (ADM).

involving different antidepressant medications, different cognitive therapists, and using different follow-up intervals, appeared to provide relatively compelling evidence that cognitive therapy, even if only used in the acute phase, could reduce the risk of future relapse. Taken together with the evidence that maintenance interpersonal therapy could reduce rates of relapse/recurrence, there could be little doubt that psychological treatments could play a major role in dealing with the increased burden of depression faced by individuals and society. Yet evidence from the studies of cognitive therapy shown in Figure 2.1 had two important implications for the chances of producing a maintenance version, the first negative, the second more positive.

First, if cognitive therapy were shown reliably to reduce rates of relapse following recovery to the level of 20–25%, then why develop a maintenance version at all? Of course, it is always possible to do better, and perhaps with some fine-tuning, relapse rates could drop even lower, perhaps to 10–15%. As we saw it, however, this was more a question of modifying the existing components of the cognitive therapy package, perhaps by adding interventions to address residual symptoms, than actually designing an intervention for depressed patients in recovery.

But, second, the data clearly implied that the practice of cognitive therapy had taught people something that, once learned, protected them against future depression. This implication was potentially of enormous significance. Recall that, up to this point, both pharmacological and psychological approaches had assumed that once a person had recovered, the best way of dealing with the risk of relapse was to extend whatever treatment he or she had already received. The words "continuation" and "maintenance" carry with them this assumption. But why should the options be so confined? Why not use one approach to deal with acute depression and another to keep people well once they have recovered?

For the first time, we began to see that this way of looking at the problem gave rise to new possibilities. If we could understand how cognitive therapy had its protective effect, we might then devise a way of teaching that "something" to people who had recovered from their depression. This could be done even if people had not had cognitive therapy when they were depressed. In particular, patients could take antidepressant medication during acute depression (and since this remained the most common treatment for depression, it seemed a sensible option), then use a maintenance version of cognitive therapy to stay well. Patients not able to take maintenance medication would be protected after recovery by learning the same principles and practices that cognitive therapy teaches to acutely depressed patients.

There were other benefits to this approach. Patients would not have to continue to take antidepressant medication indefinitely. Furthermore, such a maintenance version of cognitive therapy delivered in a group format could have tremendous advantages in cost-efficiency. It would also allow greater numbers of patients to be helped compared to standard individual cognitive therapy.

What would such a treatment look like, could it be developed, and how effective would it be? Answers to these questions would depend very much on our ability to answer two basic questions. First, what are the important psychological mechanisms involved in depressive relapse? Second, how are these modified during the course of acute cognitive therapy? Only after answering both questions could we begin to think about offering patients who had never had cognitive therapy the same type of protection. As we see later, several pointers in the research literature indicated how the first question might be answered. However, the second question remained unanswered: At that time, we simply did not know how cognitive therapy's effects reduced risk of relapse. We needed to go back to basics.

COGNITIVE VULNERABILITY TO RELAPSE AND RECURRENCE

As we have seen, one of the major contributions that the cognitive model of emotional disorders made during the 1970s and 1980s was its assertion that the way we think about ourselves, the world, and the future can have a major effect on our emotions and behavior.[44] So far, the model as we have described it only applies to the *onset* of an episode and how long it *persists* once it has established itself. Negative thinking can cause and maintain depression. But what of ongoing *vulnerability*, the risk of becoming depressed again once the person has recovered from an episode? With respect to such vulnerability, Beck proposed that, early in life, vulnerable individuals acquire certain assumptions or attitudes that persist into adulthood and become traits that endure throughout their lives.[45] When someone sees the world from such a point of view, his or her risk of suffering depression increases, because, when a negative event occurs, it is seen through the lens of the underlying belief, bringing about feelings of sadness that may be out of proportion to the event itself. In the Introduction, we mentioned briefly the questionnaire that Beck and colleagues[46] constructed as a way to measure these dysfunctional attitudes: the Dysfunctional Attitude Scale. It is now time to detail how this measure of vulnerability progressed from yielding disappointing results to intriguing and important new insights into the nature of depressive relapse.

Are Persisting Dysfunctional Attitudes the Cause of Relapse?

Items on the Dysfunctional Attitude Scale describe attitudes or assumptions that reflect, as it were, a personal contract for maintaining self-worth. As long as the conditions of the contract are met, the person is fine. If, for example, someone believes that "to be happy, I must succeed in everything I do," then his or her mood is fine so long as he or she does not fail at anything. If he or she fails an exam at college or is turned down for a promotion, the conclusion is likely "I cannot be happy" or "I cannot live with this failure." It is not hard to see how these dysfunctional attitudes were seen as enduring traits that rendered some people vulnerable to clinical depression.

What, then, did the clinical cognitive model predict about previously depressed patients' scores on the Dysfunctional Attitude Scale? Since we knew that these patients were undoubtedly vulnerable to future depression, and certainly at higher risk than people who had never been depressed, the prediction was clear. Formerly depressed patients, even if not depressed now, should have higher scores on the Dysfunctional Attitude Scale than those who had never been depressed. It was relatively easy to set up studies in which previously depressed and never-depressed participant's levels of dysfunctional attitudes were compared. Rick Ingram and colleagues recently reviewed over 40 such studies done around that time and, with very few exceptions, their conclusions were clear. Although Dysfunctional Attitude Scale scores were elevated in patients during an episode of depression, the scores of recovered patients, tested in normal mood, were not distinguishable from the scores of never-depressed people.[47] There have been few occasions in clinical psychology research in which such a strong prediction has been rejected in such a clear-cut way. Persistent dysfunctional attitudes and assumptions were not the cause of relapse.

Sad Moods Can Reawaken Negative Thoughts: A Basis for Understanding Vulnerability

If there was no good evidence for the existence of dysfunctional attitudes as persistent traits, how was vulnerability to depression to be explained cognitively? At this point, it was necessary to step back from the research on dysfunctional attitudes to consider briefly another, parallel strand of research. This other research program, begun by, among others, John Teasdale and colleagues, was not concerned with understanding the effect of thinking on mood, but with examining the other side of the vicious circle: the effect that mood has on thinking. They used experimental induction of sad moods in which participants read sad statements or listened to sad music for 5–10 minutes. The effects of the mood inductions were short-lived and reversible, lasting from 5 to 10 minutes, but provided a valuable window on the types of changes in thinking brought on by mild depression.

Several studies found that if nondepressed people were experimentally induced into mild depressed moods, then they showed negative biases in memory. They were less likely (and took longer) to recall pleasant events that had happened in their lives, and more likely to recall negative events. Previous researchers had observed such biases in clinical depression but had been inconclusive about how such biases were caused.[48,49] Depressed people might recall more negative memories simply because they had experienced more such events, or because they evaluated their whole lives as negative. The experimental work showed that the biasing effects of depression on memory were not simply the result of more negative events in depressed persons' lives. Such negative events undoubtedly occur, but, to add to the misery, depressed persons must also cope with a mood-induced bias that focuses more on negativity in their lives and less on any positive aspects.

This suggested a different way of looking at vulnerability. Perhaps the important difference between individuals who had recovered from depression and those who had never been depressed was not in how they thought about things when their moods were fine, but rather, what came to mind when they were feeling sad. Could the answer to what makes people vulnerable to future depression lie in the patterns of negative thinking previously associated with experiences of depression? We already knew some of the central symptoms of depression: guilt, remorse, and negative, self-critical thinking. During an episode of depression, people experience both depressed mood and negative thinking. What if, during an episode, there occurred a learned association between one and the other? In the future, the occurrence of just one element (mood) would bring about the other (change in thinking patterns). For people who have been depressed in the past, even normal, day-to-day sadness might have serious consequences.

John Teasdale called this the "differential activation hypothesis,"[49] the idea being that sad moods were likely to reactivate thinking styles associated with previous sad moods. These styles would differ from one individual to another, depending on individuals' past experiences. Teasdale suggested that differential accessibility could help us understand depressive relapse. Whereas most people might be able to ignore the occasional sad mood, in previously depressed persons a slight lowering of mood might bring about a large and potentially devastating change in thought patterns. These thought patterns would most often involve global, negative self-judgments such as "I am worthless" and "I am stupid."

Experiments were carried out to test these ideas. In these studies, people who were no longer depressed, but who had been depressed in the past were examined with and without mood induction. The question was: How would formerly depressed people react to experimental induction of a sad mood, and how would such a mood impact on their thinking compared to people who had never been depressed? The results from a number of such studies (reviewed by Segal and Ingram[50]) suggested that even when the sadness brought about by the experiment was similar in previously depressed and never-depressed persons, the mood had a more telling impact for those with a history of depression. People who had been depressed before showed an exaggerated cognitive bias.

The negative thinking reactivated in recovered patients would act to maintain and intensify the moods in a series of vicious cycles. In this way, in persons with a history of major depression, states of mild sadness would be more likely to progress to more intense and persistent states, increasing the risk of future onset of major depressive episodes. This very simple but powerful idea succeeded in turning attention away from measuring the levels of dysfunctional or biased thinking in nondepressed mood, and focused instead on how easily mood could reactivate this thinking.

Sad Moods Reactivate Vulnerable Attitudes and Beliefs

At the end of the 1980s, the work of Jeanne Miranda and Jackie Persons added new and important evidence. In several studies, they looked at the effects of mood, not on measures of memory, as John Teasdale had done, but on the very same measure of dysfunctional attitudes that had yielded the earlier disappointing results. They found that when never-depressed individuals reported feeling sad, their belief in such attitudes changed relatively little. By contrast, when formerly depressed patients reported feeling sad, they were more likely to endorse dysfunctional attitudes than when their moods were fine. For example, when sad, such persons were more likely to believe that, to be happy, they must succeed in everything they did.[51,52]

These findings pointed to the same conclusion that Teasdale had reached: Just a small increase in sadness, for those who had been depressed before, could lead to a reinstatement of the thinking patterns they had experienced when depressed. To use a computer analogy, the "depressive thinking" program had not really been wiped from the hard disk during recovery; small shifts in mood could reinstall it, as if it had never been absent.

Our thinking at the outset of the MacArthur project was that the degree to which people showed mood-activated reinstatement of negative thinking patterns most likely predicted relapse and recurrence in depression. A subsequent study confirmed this hypothesis. Zindel Segal and his colleagues induced a temporary sad mood in depressed patients who had just completed treatment (either antidepressants or cognitive therapy) at the Center for Addiction and Mental Health in Toronto. Their aim was to determine the effect of the treatments on dysfunctional beliefs: particularly, whether the treatments effected changes in the beliefs in response to increases in sad mood. Segal and colleagues also wanted to see how well mood-related changes on the Dysfunctional Attitude Scale predicted patients' subsequent relapse.

The results showed that those patients with the greatest increase in dysfunctional beliefs following the "mood challenge" were more likely to suffer a relapse over the subsequent 30 months.[53] Furthermore, the patients who had undergone cognitive therapy showed less reactivity: Their dysfunctional attitudes shifted less in response to the mood challenge. This was further confirmation of our rapidly forming view that such "cognitive reactivity," the tendency to react to small changes in mood with large changes in negative thinking, was the issue that had to be addressed in order to prevent depression. Furthermore, data from other sources suggested that cognitive reactivity might have a cumulative effect, with each episode of depression increasing the likelihood of yet another episode.

PATHWAYS TO RELAPSE ARE MORE EASILY ACTIVATED OVER TIME

In 1992, Robert Post,[33] an eminent biological psychiatrist, published a paper in which he suggested that, rather than remaining constant, the relationship between psychological stress and depressive relapse changes over time. He reviewed a large amount of data suggesting the need to revise our view of the link between stressful events and the onset of depression. Previous discussion of the impact of events on depression had been largely limited to whether negative life events are sufficient to cause the onset of depression, or whether they need to occur in combination (or interaction) with other vulnerability factors. The data reviewed by Post suggested a more complex picture. *Early* episodes of depression were, indeed, often preceded by significant negative events. However, as more episodes of depression were experienced, stressful events played a progressively less important role. It seemed that later episodes of depression were more and more easily triggered (see Figure 2.2). Post argued that each new episode contributes to small changes in the neurobiological

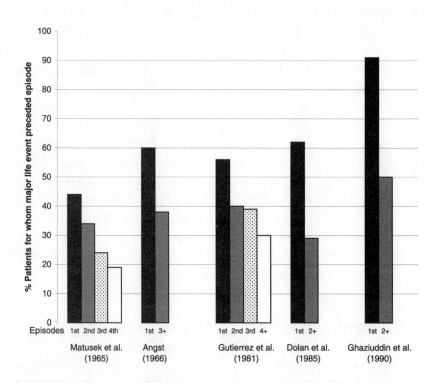

FIGURE 2.2. Studies of the link between stressful life events and first versus subsequent episodes for depression. Data from Post.[33] See Post for references to studies reviewed.

threshold at which depression can be triggered, and that, with time, this threshold is lowered to the point that episodes seem to occur spontaneously, as if independent of circumstances in the person's life. Although he had been working within a neurobiological understanding of depression, his ideas were very consistent with our view that repeated episodes of depression could make the psychological processes involved in the onset of a new episode more autonomous.[54]

THE RUMINATIVE MIND

Let us take stock for a moment. We have seen that persistence of "dysfunctional" ways of looking at the world cannot explain why some people remain vulnerable to future depression. When depressed people recover, their view of the world appears, on the face of it, to be restored to normal. In any event, it resembles the view of someone who has never been depressed. But despite this apparent normality, depression leaves its mark. What remains, once depression is over, is a tendency to react to small changes in mood with large changes in negative thinking.

Note that, up to now, we have focused on the way mood can bring to mind certain types of thoughts, memories, beliefs, and so on. We have, as it were, focused on the *contents* of consciousness. But there was also increasing evidence that people who are vulnerable to depression differ from other people in the *way* they deal with depressed mood itself.

Susan Nolen-Hoeksema, in a number of important studies, has shown that there are marked differences in people's reactions to depressive moods and situations. Some people respond to low mood by acting in ways that focus attention on themselves, while others do things that take their minds away from themselves. Nolen-Hoeksema refers to the first way of reacting as the "ruminative response style," and assesses people's tendency to react in this way with her Response Styles Questionnaire, which asks people to indicate how often they think or do a number of things when they feel down, sad, or depressed; for example, "Analyze recent events to try and understand why you are depressed" or "Think about how passive and unmotivated you feel." People who ruminate in this way tend to prolong sad feelings. By contrast, others are less likely to ruminate, and many engage in activities that allow them to distract themselves from such feelings. Such tendencies are assessed by the Distraction subscale of the Response Styles Questionnaire; for example, "Try to find something positive in the situation or something you learned" or "Do something you enjoy." People who tend to use such distraction techniques are more likely to experience more short-lived depressed moods.

A dramatic illustration of the importance of the ruminative response style came from a study conducted by Susan Nolen-Hoeksema and her colleagues.[55] This study took advantage of the fact that they had assessed people on their measure of ruminative response style shortly before the 1989 Loma Prieta earthquake in California. They found that people who reported (before the earthquake occurred) a tendency to respond to depression by ruminating had the highest depression scores following the earthquake.

One of the problems of research that finds an association between a cognitive trait, such as ruminative response style on the one hand, and depression on the other, is that we can never be sure that the depression is not being caused by a third factor (e.g., another personality trait, such as neuroticism) that simply correlates with ruminative tendencies. There is a way out of this difficulty, however. It is possible to mimic the effects of different cognitive styles in the laboratory, and to examine their impact on mood. In this case, Nolen-Hoeksema and her colleagues carried out experiments in which nondepressed college students were given a mood induction procedure and then randomly allocated to one of two conditions. In the first condition, they were given instructions to think about themselves, and why they were the way they were (the "rumination" condition). In the second condition, they were instructed to think about things unrelated to themselves (the "distraction" condition). Results showed that the mood induction produced more persistent and intense sadness in the rumination group.

This sort of experiment can also address other important aspects of rumination. For example, why does rumination persist if it does so much damage? When asked why they chose to ruminate about their feelings in this way, many people said that they believed it would give them a better understanding of their emotions, and that this would help them solve their problems.[56] Using an experimental approach, Lyubomirsky and Nolen-Hoeksema found that the opposite was true. They asked people either to ruminate about, or to distract themselves from, their sad mood, and then assessed subjects' ability to solve problems by using the Means–Ends Problem Solving task. This widely used task gives participants the beginning of a story about a problematic situation (e.g., a relationship breakup) with a "happy ending." Participants complete the story to say how the problem was solved. The results of this study revealed a dramatic contrast between belief and reality. Participants who ruminated about their mood *believed* they understood themselves better but actually showed a reduction, rather than an improvement, in their ability to solve problems.

With Nolen-Hoeksema's findings, and the work comparing depression-induced negative thinking in recovered depressed and never-depressed people, we now had two important approaches to what makes people psychologically vulnerable to depression: First, the relatively easy accessibility of negative material (thoughts, memories, attitudes) when mood is low; second, the way some people handle such negative moods and material by ruminating about them. Which approach should be chosen, or could both play a role? In the end, it turned out that these were not alternatives. In reality, they were two aspects of an entire "package" of changes brought about by depression. Let us take a particular example to illustrate this.

Imagine the following situation: Mary has just returned from work, tired and looking forward to a relaxing evening watching television. A message on the answering machine indicates her partner will be late coming home. She feels disappointed, angry, and upset. She brings to mind other occasions earlier in the month, when the same thing happened. A thought about possible unfaithfulness comes to mind. She dismisses the thought, but it returns with greater vividness as she imagines that she heard some laughter in the background on the taped message. She feels nauseated. But it does not end there. With increasing speed, her mind conjures up images of the possible future: separating, seeing lawyers, getting divorced, buying another place, living in poverty. She can feel herself getting more upset as anger turns to depression and she recalls episodes in the past when she was rejected and alone. She "knows" that all their mutual friends probably would not want to know *her* anymore. Tears well up in Mary's eyes and she is left wondering what she can do. She decides to go for a walk and try to work out why it is that she always reacts this way.

Note the avalanche of feelings, thoughts, and bodily sensations here. But note also that it is not just the negative material that causes Mary to be upset, nor is it simply the *way* she deals with material. Rather, it seems as if a whole mode of mind, a configuration or pattern of negative mood/thoughts/images/body sensations, has been "wheeled into place" in response to this situation. This mode of mind includes *both* the easily accessible negative material *and* the tendency to deal with it by ruminating. But it also includes feedback loops involving the effects of emotion on the body.

People in such a state of mind spend a good deal of their time ruminating about why they feel the way they do and trying to understand their problems and personal inadequacies. They believe that thinking about things in this way should help them find ways to reduce their distress, but the method they use to achieve that aim is actually counterproductive. In fact, in this state of mind, repeatedly "thinking about" negative aspects of the self, or of problematic situations, serves to perpetuate rather than to resolve depression.

We wrote up these "best guesses" about the causes of vulnerability to depression in a paper in *Behaviour Research and Therapy*.[57] What we believed was happening to cognitively vulnerable people was as follows: At times of lowering mood, old, habitual patterns of cognitive processing switch in relatively automatically. This has two important effects. First, thinking runs repeatedly around fairly well-worn "mental grooves," without finding an effective way forward out of depression. Second, this thinking, itself, intensifies depressed mood, which in turn leads to further thoughts. In this way, through self-perpetuating vicious cycles, otherwise mild and transient mood can escalate into more severe and disabling depressed states (as summarized in Figure 2.3). We have more to say in Chapter 4 about this model, and its effect on our understanding of how we might take a

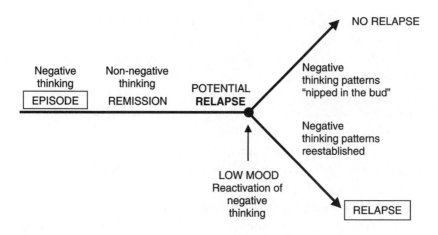

FIGURE 2.3. A sketch of the model underlying the development of mindfulness-based cognitive therapy for prevention of depressive relapse/recurrence.

radically different approach to reducing the risk of relapse. As we saw it, the task of relapse prevention is to help patients disengage from these ruminative and self-perpetuating modes of mind when they feel sad, or at other times of potential relapse. With this model of vulnerability in our minds, we could return to the question of how cognitive therapy achieves its effects.

HOW DOES COGNITIVE THERAPY REDUCE RELAPSE AND RECURRENCE IN DEPRESSION?

Although, by the late 1980s, there had been studies showing that cognitive therapy reduces risk of relapse, nobody knew how it had this effect. As we have seen, the original clinical model underlying cognitive therapy for depression suggested that vulnerability to depression is related to the persistence of certain underlying dysfunctional attitudes or assumptions. From this perspective, reduction in risk of relapse following cognitive therapy would be seen as the result of specific effects of cognitive therapy in reducing those dysfunctional attitudes. This hypothesis received little empirical support.[58] In studies in which cognitive therapy produced significantly better long-term outcomes than pharmacotherapy, the two treatments often did not differ on posttreatment measures of dysfunctional thinking (Dysfunctional Attitude Scale).[59] This extremely important finding reinforces the view that the *level* of such attitudes, when people are not depressed, is not the point at issue.

What then were the cognitive processes through which cognitive therapy reduced relapse and recurrence in depression? At the time that we considered this central question, it was generally assumed that cognitive therapy, which primarily targets changing belief in depressive thoughts and dysfunctional attitudes, had its effects through changes in the *content* of depressive thinking. Our more detailed theoretical analysis suggested a different possibility.[57] Although the explicit emphasis in cognitive therapy is on changing thought content, we realized that it was equally possible that when successful, this treatment led implicitly to changes in patients' *relationships* to their negative thoughts and feelings. Specifically, as a result of repeatedly identifying negative thoughts as they arose and standing back from them to evaluate the accuracy of their content, patients often made a more general shift in their *perspective* on negative thoughts and feelings. Rather than regarding thoughts as necessarily true or as an aspect of the self, patients switched to a perspective within which negative thoughts and feelings could be seen as passing events in the mind that were neither necessarily valid reflections of reality nor central aspects of the self. The importance of such "distancing" or "decentering" had previously been recognized in discussions of cognitive therapy,[18] but usually as a means to an end, changing thought content, rather than an end in itself.

Others, however, had suggested a more central role for decentering. Rick Ingram and Steve Hollon[60] suggested that "cognitive therapy relies heavily on helping individuals switch to a controlled mode of processing that is metacognitive in nature and focuses on depression-related cognition . . . typically referred to as 'distancing' . . . the long-term effectiveness of cognitive therapy may lie in teaching patients to initiate this process in the face of future stress" (p. 272).

This alternative perspective on how cognitive therapy might produce its effects represented a fundamental shift in our understanding. Previously, we, and others, had seen decentering as one of a number of things going on in cognitive therapy. Our analysis suggested that it was central. As we conceived it then, decentering meant seeing thoughts in a wider perspective, sufficient to be able to see them as simply "thoughts" rather than necessarily reflecting reality. This fundamental aspect of cognitive therapy protected people against future depression. If such decentering did not take place, patients would be left arguing with themselves about whether their thoughts were true or not, marshaling evidence for or against a negative thought, and at risk of simply getting caught up in the thought pattern.

The shift gave us the freedom to consider alternative approaches to relapse prevention. The task was to find ways to teach people to decenter from their negative thoughts; preferably in a way that would take up the cognitive "space" in a mind otherwise filled with ruminative thoughts. (We have not said much about this aspect of the model, for it will take us too far afield. Suffice it to say that most models of mind assume that conscious, aware forms of information processing take up space in a "limited capacity channel." This implies that if the limited channel can be filled with nonruminative material, the person, for that period, will simply be unable to ruminate. See Teasdale et al.[57] for more details of this aspect of our thinking.)

Could we get at these processes directly? That is, could we find a way to bring about a shift in a person's relationship to his or her negative thoughts and feelings, in a way that would have no elements explicitly directed at changing thought content? At this point, luck intervened, for one of our colleagues had also been considering similar issues with her patients.

Marsha Linehan had spent part of her 1991 sabbatical leave with John Teasdale and Mark Williams at the Medical Research Council's Applied Psychology Unit in Cambridge. She had used the concept of decentering in her development of dialectical behavior therapy.[61] She had worked many years developing this psychological treatment for people who presented clinicians with some of their most challenging problems: those with a diagnosis of "borderline personality disorder." This disorder is characterized by, among other things, many attempts at self-harm, unstable emotions, intolerance of being alone, unstable relationships, and sometimes abnormal "dissociative" experiences.

Her view of the role of changing the relationship to negative thoughts and feelings in psychological treatment was to provide patients with more options for how they might choose to respond to an event, rather than just be carried away by the experience itself. In the treatment manual she developed, numerous exercises trained patients to pay attention to their experience in ways that allowed them to observe events as they were occurring. She maintained that, in order to attend to an event, we usually need to be able to step back from it. For example, "walking" and "observing walking" are two different things.[62] She had introduced a training procedure called "mindfulness" in the service of helping her patients protect themselves from their more powerful thoughts and emotions, by showing them how to step back from them and relate to them less literally.

While in Cambridge, Linehan had been working on an *Archives of General Psychiatry* article reporting the results of her clinical trial[61] and had talked about the use of such mindfulness meditation in her treatment. She had mentioned the name of Jon Kabat-Zinn in Worcester, Massachusetts, who had been exploring the use of mindfulness in a health care setting with patients suffering from chronic pain. Now, over a year after that sabbatical conversation, in looking for ways to help train recovered depressed patients to deal with depressive thinking triggered by sad moods, we wondered whether we ought to look closely at the work of Jon Kabat-Zinn.

MINDFULNESS

Marsha Linehan had powerfully argued the case for including mindfulness as a possible component of psychological treatment. But what is meant by "mindfulness"? We looked at Jon Kabat-Zinn's definition: "Mindfulness means paying attention in a particular way: on purpose, in the present moment, and nonjudgmentally" (p. 4).[63] This was remarkable in its directness and simplicity. How was mindfulness used in practice? Jon Kabat-Zinn's Stress Reduction Clinic at the University of Massachusetts (UMass) Medical Center had several unique features. In it, he taught participants the ancient practice of mindfulness meditation, adapted from its use as a spiritual practice to extend its availability and relevance to patients suffering from a variety of chronic physical illnesses. His aim was to equip patients with ways of responding to the stress in their lives that allowed them to step out of those mental reactions that often worsened the stress and interfered with effective problem solving.

The accounts of what his patients were getting out of the program bore a striking similarity to what we were beginning to see as the central change process in cognitive therapy. It became rapidly clear when we started to read about mindfulness-based stress reduction (MBSR) how mindfulness fostered a decentered relationship to mental contents by training people to take a wider perspective, in order to observe their thinking as it was occurring. The way Jon Kabat-Zinn expressed this could not have summed up more accurately what we had in mind when we were trying to understand how cognitive therapy had its decentering effects: "It is remarkable how liberating it feels to be able to see that your thoughts are just thoughts and that they are not 'you' or 'reality.' . . . . the simple act of recognizing your thoughts as thoughts can free you from the distorted reality they often create and allow for more clear-sightedness and a greater sense of manageability in your life" (pp. 69–70).[64] This most significant element struck a chord with us at that time.

For example, there is a story in *Full Catastrophe Living* (the book that describes the MBSR program[64]) about a patient who had just recovered from a heart attack. He found himself washing his car in his driveway at 10 o'clock at night, using floodlights for illumination! All of a sudden, he had the realization that he didn't have to be doing this. The idea that he must wash his car was just a thought. It was just that he never stopped to question what he thought needed doing.

There were a number of other reasons to believe that this approach might be relevant. First, the mindfulness practice Jon Kabat-Zinn taught to his patients involved exercises in awareness. According to our understanding of the factors that allow the thought–affect cycles to self-perpetuate, any exercise in purposeful awareness would have the advantage of "taking up capacity" in the limited information processing channel. This would starve the vicious ruminative cycles of the resources needed to maintain them.

Second, such practice at becoming aware of thoughts, feelings, and bodily sensations might meet the need we had identified to help patients recognize at an early stage the times they were most likely to slide into depression. Mindfulness exercises might provide an early warning system of an impending avalanche, so that it could be stopped before the rocks started to slide.

Third, we could not ignore a further aspect of the MBSR program at UMass: classes of 30 or more people at a time. Here was an approach that promised to meet the larger need of an increasing number of patients suffering from depression. And all this took place in a context where no attempt was made to deal with the particular content of any individual's thoughts.

Here was another way to reach the same end of decentering that we considered critical to the relapse prevention effects of cognitive therapy. MBSR was a fully developed and highly cost-efficient treatment program, with good empirical support, that could be made available to many patients. Could we use this as a template in developing our own approach with recovered depressed patients? While these skills had not been shown to be applicable to problems in clinically depressed patients, there was encouraging evidence for their efficacy in related disorders that often went along with depression (e.g., chronic pain,[66] generalized anxiety disorder[65]). There was also evidence that some form of mindfulness practice was maintained on a regular basis by a majority of patients up to 3 years after the initial training had been completed.[67]

In summary, mindfulness appeared to offer a number of possibilities for approaching relapse prevention. We saw it as providing alternative methods for teaching decentering skills, training patients to recognize when their mood was deteriorating, and using techniques that would take up limited resources in channels of information processing that normally sustained ruminative thought–affect cycles.

MAKING CONTACT
WITH THE STRESS REDUCTION CLINIC
AT UMASS MEDICAL CENTER

So why, then, did we not rush to Worcester, Massachusetts, and embrace these ideas? We discussed the possibility of contacting Dr. Kabat-Zinn but we could not easily agree on whether this was a good idea. There were reasons to be cautious. For one thing, such an exploration of mindfulness and awareness training would take us away from our brief to design a maintenance form of cognitive therapy. Furthermore, only one of us had experience with meditation practice, on the basis of which he believed it might hold promise for patients who had been depressed. But we also had to recognize a more skeptical view. What evidence was there that mindfulness meditation was any more effective than relaxation training? Hadn't Peter McLean's study in 1979 shown the unequivocal superiority of cognitive-behavioral therapy over relaxation in treating depression?[68] And if we were attracted because of its affinity with cognitive therapy principles and practice, why not stay with cognitive therapy? Finally, we must admit that we were unsure how such a move might affect our scientific colleagues. Meditation seemed too close to a form of religious practice, and though each of us had a different "take" on religion, we all felt that such personal issues were best left outside the lab and the clinic.

So, although there were many reasons for exploring mindfulness further, we had many reservations. We agreed in the end that we would at least explore further the mindfulness approach. We would contact Dr. Kabat-Zinn and pilot-test some of the mindfulness exercises with one or two patients. At this stage, it was not clear which way the project would go. Differences of opinion can be seen in the different tone of two letters sent the very same day. The first was sent by Zindel Segal to John Teasdale; the second, by John Teasdale to Jon Kabat-Zinn. Only when we went through our own archives to prepare this book did we noticed the curious juxtaposition of attitudes.

Zindel Segal's letter betrays an uneasy tone:

. . . I have had the opportunity to try out the "just pay attention to your breathing" technique with a patient who is 6 months post-depression. Her reaction was generally receptive and she agreed to keep a log for a month and practice "observing her attention wander and return to her thoughts." My reaction, on the other hand, is that I was teaching her to meditate!!!, and this made me feel somewhat uncomfortable. It will be interesting to compare notes in January . . .

John Teasdale's letter was very different. It is explicit in its enthusiasm about exploring this new territory:

. . . given the apparent importance of streams of negative thoughts in the maintenance of clinical depression, I have become increasingly interested in the possible use of meditation-related procedures . . .

And

I have been very impressed by your ability to extract the essence of Buddhist mindfulness meditation and to translate it into a format that is accessible and clearly very effective in helping the average U.S. citizen. For both personal and professional reasons, I would very much like to explore the applicability of your work to treatment of depression.

Our collective mix of enthusiasm and curiosity on the one hand, and diffidence and alarm on the other, might not be atypical of the reactions of other behaviorally and cognitively trained therapists. Despite a good degree of skepticism and differences among us, it was clear from reading and listening to the tapes used in the program that MBSR included at least some elements that might be very helpful to the maintenance version of cognitive therapy we still expected to develop. We wanted to see firsthand what actual skills patients were learning in MBSR, whatever the philosophy behind their delivery.

We now had a theoretical model that emphasized the importance of changing patient's relationships to their negative thoughts and feelings. We had moved away from thinking that the key ingredient in cognitive therapy (the reason why it had such long-lasting effects) was that it changed a person's degree of belief in his or her thoughts and attitudes. Instead, we believed that the key was whether people could learn to take a decentered perspective on their patterns of thinking. If this were true, then there was no need to change the content of people's thoughts, but only how they related to this content. We had recognized that, in the MBSR program, there appeared to be an emphasis on decentering from which we might learn. We visited Jon Kabat-Zinn in October, 1993, to sit in on a number of his classes.

CHAPTER 3

⊗

Developing Mindfulness-Based Cognitive Therapy

Jon Kabat-Zinn set up the Stress Reduction Clinic (offering mindfulness-based stress reduction [MBSR]) at the University of Massachusetts Medical Center, in Worcester, Massachusetts, in the 1970s. Since then, he and his colleagues have helped more than 10,000 people with a range of conditions, including heart disease, cancer, AIDS, chronic pain, stress-related gastrointestinal problems, headaches, high blood pressure, sleep disorders, anxiety, and panic. By 1993, the clinic had already evaluated the efficacy of its approach with patients suffering from anxiety disorders[65] and chronic pain.[66] The evidence showed that most participants experienced long-lasting physical and psychological symptom reduction, as well as deep positive changes in attitude, behavior, and perception of self, others, and the world.

What does the stress reduction clinic at Massachusetts actually do? The program consists of eight weekly 2½-hour sessions, at which instructors meet with around 30 patients. Patients are seen individually a few days or weeks before the program starts. At that meeting, time is taken to talk to prospective participants about their past, their current concerns, and what they hope to get out of the program. The nature of the classes is explained, including the fact that taking the stress reduction classes may be stressful! The program involves a great deal of commitment. For example, daily homework exercises (lasting up to an hour a day) are an essential element of the program.

Once a person has started the program, the primary work is intensive training in mindfulness meditation. The aim is to increase patients' awareness of present, moment-to-moment, experience. They receive extensive practice in learning to bring their attention back to the present, using a focus on the breath as an "anchor," whenever they notice that their attention has been diverted to streams of thought, worries, or general lack of awareness.

FIRST IMPRESSIONS

On our first visit to the Stress Reduction Clinic, we were invited to sit in on Session 1 of the MBSR program led by Jon Kabat-Zinn. The classes were held in a large, carpeted conference room. The first thing we noticed was that the composition of the group was different from what we were accustomed to, in that many patients appeared to be dealing with very difficult medical conditions. Although we knew that the clinic had been originally set up to deal with severe and chronic physical illness and disability, it remained unclear whether the experience would be relevant to relapse in depression as we had thought.

The theme of the first class focused on becoming more aware of the tendency we all have to be on automatic pilot much of the time; how we do ordinary things (such as eating) in everyday life, without really being aware of what we are doing. Later on, the instructor led the class through an exercise that involved taking awareness to different parts of the body in turn (the "body scan"). The instruction was simply to be aware, moment by moment, of sensations in each part of the body, rather than trying to alter them in any way.

Although the contents of the session were different, nothing appeared inconsistent with our own methods in cognitive therapy. In fact, the emphasis on being more aware of things, of stepping out of automatic pilot, was central to our view that people who had been depressed needed to learn to be more aware of the early warning signals indicating times when their mood might deteriorate. Here were some exercises that might help them do just that.

The program builds on the initial experience with the body scan, introducing in later sessions meditation on the breath, the body, sights, and sounds. More attention is paid to body sensations than is common in most psychological treatments for depression, using yoga stretches and mindful walking to explore, in some detail, different aspects of feelings as they might be expressed in bodily sensations.

It was clear from the outset that the MBSR program utilized a psychoeducational model. Its stress reduction techniques, such as focusing on breathing or yoga stretches, are those that many people choose to do in their spare time as a way to promote health and well-being. But in addition, participants are taught, whatever their chosen focus of attention at any moment, to allow, as best they can, thoughts, feelings, and sensations to come and go in the mind. The instruction is to notice how the mind often tends to become attached to an experience judged to be positive, and avoids or escapes an experience judged to be negative. In addition to noting this in daily practice, at one point in the course, participants are given homework in which they keep a diary of pleasant and (a week later) unpleasant events. They are asked to pay special attention to thoughts, feelings, and body sensations associated with each event they record.

After the first class, subsequent sessions start with practice (that is, the instructor leads the class in a meditation such as a body scan, or a sitting meditation with focus on the breath). The remainder of each session mixes dialogue, further practice, poetry, story, and awareness exercises, all in the service of helping participants become more aware of the "here and now" (for details, see Kabat-Zinn's *Full Catastrophe Living*[64]). The basic message of the program is that we all (whether patients or clinicians) frequently find ourselves swept away by the currents of thought and feeling related to the past, present, or future. We often lose the vividness of the present moment by "being somewhere else." When we are able to be in the present moment, we become more awake in our lives, more aware of each moment, more aware of the choices open to us.

Although some of the vocabulary used in the stress reduction program was not what we would normally use in cognitive therapy, it appeared to us from our first visit, together with our reading about the program and listening to its tapes, that we could relatively easily combine the two approaches without having to make too many changes in the way we worked with patients. We were particularly attracted to the fact that patients in the program learn generic skills of attentional control. Because these skills are generic, learning does not depend on the presence of negative thoughts and feelings. They can be practiced on a wide range of experiences in everyday life. This looked as if it would suit our purposes very well, for we wanted a procedure that could be used when patients were not currently feeling depressed. At this point, patients would be looking for something to increase positive well-being and perhaps reduce the risk of future depression, rather than something to reduce current symptoms of depression.

Furthermore, participants in MBSR are asked to practice mindfulness skills on a daily basis as part of their homework, and the evidence suggested that they continued to do this long after they had completed the MBSR program (up to 3 years[67]). This seemed to be a valuable way to keep new learning active, so it was very relevant to depressed patients in recovery, whose task is to remain prepared for an event that might not happen until months, or even years, later. If patients ran into difficulties, the daily practice ensured that the skills could be recalled and implemented more easily. In addition, it seemed to us that practice in increased awareness of momentary experience made it more likely that patients would detect at the earliest possible stage any signs of incipient relapse. Patients would therefore be more likely to take appropriate action at a point when interventions have the greatest chance of success. We began to see how we might design a program that, in combining MBSR and cognitive therapy into a new form of cognitive therapy, would help recovered depressed patients stay well.

REASONS TO BE CAUTIOUS

In that first visit, the instructors at UMass sounded a note of caution. If we were serious about incorporating mindfulness in our approach, then, as prospective instructors, we would have to have our own mindfulness meditation practice. Frankly, we were not at all sure

about this. After all, we did not intend to teach MBSR, but to incorporate some of their techniques into our maintenance form of cognitive therapy. We were interested mainly in the theoretical and
practical convergence we could see between mindfulness and cognitive approaches: the need to notice warning signs earlier; the
need to decenter from negative thoughts; the need to deploy attention in ways that would starve the self-perpetuating, relapse-related
thought–affect cycles of cognitive resources. None of this seemed to
require us to develop a mindfulness meditation practice. So we simply "took note" of their opinion on the issue: We could think about
that later.

We had seen enough on our first visit to confirm our view that
MBSR might be a convenient vehicle to teach many of the principles
and practices of decentering, and to bring about a reduction in risk of
relapse. Of course, we had only witnessed Session 1, but given that
we had, at that time, a pretty definite view of what changes had to be
brought about in formerly depressed patients, we could easily imagine that the remainder of the sessions (if we had time to sit in on
them) would also confirm our view.

As it was, we decided to incorporate mindfulness into a "regular"
cognitive therapy format—a format that would incorporate the problem-solving approach with which we were familiar. This seemed a
good compromise. It allowed us to avoid having to adopt wholesale
the values and practices associated with meditation. And there was
much in the MBSR program we could use.

However, there was a second reason to be cautious. Combining
cognitive therapy with another, different approach (no matter how
similar) was not what we had been funded to do. Incorporating any
MBSR techniques might be construed as changing cognitive therapy
too much to qualify as simply a maintenance version of the therapy.
Furthermore, we felt that we needed an approach that could be
taught to patients who had never had cognitive therapy at the acute
stage of their depression. What we were suggesting represented a
move away from a standard maintenance therapy (i.e., a therapy that
extended the acute phase of treatment into the maintenance phase),
toward an approach that might have wider applicability, but this was

not what we had been asked to develop by the MacArthur Foundation.

It was unclear how best to proceed, and in the end, we decided to face the issue head on and contact David Kupfer to discuss the dilemma and find out what the MacArthur Foundation might think of this new plan. His decision was to be an important turning point in the project, for he encouraged us to develop whatever treatment we thought most effective. In his mind, one of the operational definitions of success was that whatever form of preventive treatment we developed be judged credible enough to secure further national funding to support its evaluation once our MacArthur monies ran out. Over the next few weeks and months, we drew up a preliminary manual of a treatment that combined some MBSR and cognitive therapy strategies, and began to draft grant applications to support its evaluation.

ATTENTIONAL CONTROL TRAINING

In order better to reflect the central role played by attentional training in our preventive intervention, we decided to call our version of cognitive therapy attentional control training. The aim of attentional control training was to combine mindfulness and cognitive approaches to enable patients to increase their awareness. This would have three positive consequences. First, awareness would enable patients to notice when they were about to undergo dangerous mood swings. Second, awareness itself would take up those scarce processing resources that might have been supporting rumination, thereby weakening it. Third, patients could then decenter or exit from the more automatic depression-linked patterns of thought that these moods habitually brought to mind. At that point, techniques from cognitive therapy could allow patients to deal with the negative thoughts that any sad moods might reactivate.

This sounded great in theory, but we needed to check these ideas out. Would the treatment be useful to our patients, and would the rationale be compelling to our academic colleagues? In relation to the first issue, we decided that we would each run our own pilot group. In relation to the second, we would send our draft treatment manual to the MacArthur Research Network for their comments.

For our pilot classes, we used the 8-week group structure developed at the Stress Reduction Clinic at UMass as the basis of attentional control training and modified it to deal with themes of preventing depressive relapse (though shortening the length of each session to 2 hours). We taught mindfulness by having the class listen to a 20-minute audiotape of mindfulness instructions by Jon Kabat-Zinn that we had shortened for the purpose. We asked participants to listen to the tape once a day as homework. The pilot groups also watched an episode of the television program *Healing from Within* (one of the Bill Moyers series, *Healing and the Mind,* produced by the Public Broadcasting Service), which featured the 8-week MBSR program conducted at the Stress Reduction Clinic.

The feedback we received from the 8-week pilot program was very revealing. Some of the patients in each group appeared to do well. It was as if they learned the skills and used them effectively to deal with problems in their lives. Other patients, however, experienced considerable difficulty in applying the skills of attentional control and observation to their emotional upheaval. To be honest, this outcome may have reflected a number of silent assumptions on our part. Reflecting now on how we ran those groups, it was as if we believed that this approach would be OK for mildly negative thoughts and feelings, but not for more severe and persistent ones. In our pilot classes, any suggestions we made to participants to increase awareness of difficult issues were politely refused. We withdrew the suggestions quickly, for we had little confidence that we could deal with such difficulties using this approach.

Our intention was that participants gradually acquire the skills of decentering, so they might subsequently use them when at risk of their thoughts and feelings spiraling out of control. But participants' experiences and behavior did not fit our carefully constructed plans. They may have recovered from depression, but they wanted to bring to the discussion the many ups and downs in their lives. The problem was that patients were looking for help in dealing with these unwanted emotions early in the program, before they had time to learn the skills of decentering and thought answering that we saw as crucial.

So how were we to respond to this situation? Recall that our main intent behind attentional control training was to teach patients skills for decentering, which would allow them to step out of the "automatic pilot" state of mind or mode, in order to nip in the bud the escalation of self-sustaining patterns of depressive thought. But what do you do when patients have emotional ups and down that cannot be dealt with by decentering from thoughts alone? What do you do when patients have tried to decenter and the negative feelings are still there? We had assumed that we would naturally move into a cognitive therapy mode for dealing with these concerns.

However, with a group of 10 or more patients, there never seemed to be enough time for the instructor to deal with everyone's problems. To handle these problems with the same thoroughness as individual cognitive therapy would normally involve identifying negative thoughts feeding unwanted emotions, considering evidence for and against such thoughts, reviewing alternative possibilities, setting behavioral experiments, and so on. Although some therapists had developed cognitive therapy in a group format, we wanted to teach other skills, too, and along with standard cognitive strategies, there was simply not enough time to do both adequately. The skills in attentional control, which were crucial to the decentering we wanted to teach participants, seemed not to be deliverable in the format we had envisioned.

Something was not quite right, but what was it? The theoretical perspective we had brought to the problem of relapse seemed coherent. Equally, the changes we had made in aspects of MBSR as we incorporated them into attentional control training seemed harmless enough. For example, we had chosen to use 20-minute audiotapes because we were not completely confident that patients would listen to longer tapes. At UMass the tapes are 40–45 minutes long. But it did not seem very plausible that these kinds of procedural changes could explain all our difficulties. It seemed that something more fundamental was amiss.

These difficulties in implementing the attentional control training program were not our only problem. We had sent a draft version of the manual to David Kupfer for his comments in the winter of 1994. He sent it out for review. To our chagrin, the review of our work was skeptical of its contribution. The concerns raised were that we focused too much on mindfulness training, leaving out the valuable cognitive therapy–based components that patients really needed. The review concluded that while the "emphasis on discrete exercises and homework-based practice would provide effective learning experiences, it is still unclear how the mindfulness techniques contribute to controlling the risk of future depressive disorder." The very thing we thought was innovative failed to impress them as being relevant at all.

At this point, we felt ourselves to be at a crossroads. We had worked hard to bring in new ideas to define the challenges faced by depressed patients in recovery and the types of interventions that would address them more directly. In spite of this, however, we had clearly not convinced this reviewer that anything new was necessary. He or she saw in our proposals only a weakening of accepted cognitive-behavioral principles and practice. In retrospect, the reviewer was right. In our first draft manual, there were possibly too few cognitive and behavioral techniques. If the patients were not going to be taught cognitive therapy skills, then there was the danger that they would be left in no-man's-land, between a therapy that had proven effectiveness in reducing relapse and a new set of principles and practices that, for depression, were dangerously unproven. We had to make a decision: Either go back to the original plan to draw up a maintenance version of cognitive therapy to be used by patients when they were well, or make much clearer the potential of the clinical implementation of the mindfulness-based approach.

WHAT WERE THE INSTRUCTORS IN MINDFULNESS-BASED STRESS REDUCTION ACTUALLY DOING?

We arrived at the Stress Reduction Clinic at UMass Medical Center for the second time in the spring of 1995, with fewer certainties. But there was another important difference. In our first visit, we had seen the first session of one class and had only talked (and read) about the remainder of the program. On this second visit, we had the chance to sit in on three different classes that were midway through the program, a time when participants were working with difficult physical and emotional issues. We now saw differences between attentional control training and the MBSR mindfulness approach that we had not seen before. In particular, we saw how experienced mindfulness teachers like Saki Santorelli, Ferris Urbanowski, and Elana Rosenbaum worked with participants' painful affects. They did not try and fix or give solutions to problems raised. When patients said they felt sad, afraid, or that they had judgmental or hopeless thoughts, they were simply encouraged to bring these difficulties to awareness and to breathe with them.

This was more than a problem of fine-tuning attentional control training. These instructors were teaching a radically different approach that encouraged participants to "allow" difficult thoughts and feelings simply to be there, to bring to them a kindly awareness, to adopt toward them a more "welcome" than a "need to solve" stance. In order to proceed any further, it was vital that we understand the nature of this difference. Without it, our attempts to integrate cognitive therapy and MBSR meaningfully would likely stop there.

Instead of translating into cognitive therapy what we saw in MBSR, we decided to look again at all aspects of MBSR, rather than just at those parts that fit our preexisting theory. We thought again about the fact that all the MBSR instructors were themselves practicing mindfulness meditation, and that they seemed able to embody the same gentle approach to patients' difficulties that the patients themselves were being encouraged to take. The stance of the instructor was itself "invitational." In addition, there was always the assumption of "continuity" between the experiences of the instructor and the participants. If class members described becoming aware of how they had been criticizing themselves, for example, the experience of dealing with self-critical thoughts was something the instructor had in common with others in the class. The assumption here was simple: that minds tend to operate in similar ways, and there is no basis for

discriminating between the minds of those seeking help and those offering it.

As we contemplated this change, we became aware of an issue
that we could not put off any longer: our own mindfulness practice.
Recall that when we first visited the Stress Reduction Clinic and
started our pilot work, we had seen MBSR as mostly a vehicle for
teaching participants attentional control as a skills training exercise.
We felt that the technique could be adequately conveyed using the
audiotapes of Jon Kabat-Zinn's meditation instructions both in class
and for homework. This view ran counter to the spirit of the message
we were getting from the staff at the Stress Reduction Clinic.

The staff at the Stress Reduction Clinic had consistently emphasized the importance of instructors having their own meditation
practice, and within minutes of first meeting us, they asked about our
personal commitment to the practice of mindfulness. We had now
seen for ourselves the remarkable way they were able to embody a
different relationship to the most intense distress and emotion in
their patients. And we had seen the MBSR instructors going further
in their work with negative affect than we had been able to do in the
group context, by staying within our therapist roles. We now saw
more clearly how these two things were connected: that this ability to
relate differently to negative affect came from having their own ongoing mindfulness practice, so that they might teach mindfulness out of
their experience of it. A vital part of what the MBSR instructor conveyed was his or her own embodiment of mindfulness in interactions
with the class.

This ultimately persuaded us of the wisdom of the advice we had
not wholly heeded on our first visit. Participants in the MBSR program
learn about mindfulness in two ways: through their own practice, and
when the instructor him- or herself is able to embody it in the way issues are dealt with in the class. This was different from our earlier con-
ception of mindfulness as a technique in which patients could be
trained by a therapist who might or might not have been mindful him-
or herself. If the therapists themselves are not mindful as they teach,
the extent to which class members can learn mindfulness will be limited. Just as in rock climbing, those who are learning need to feel that

the instructor has both the skill and experience to deal with the difficult situations that will arise. In the same way, mindfulness training involves the instructor participating alongside the patient, not giving instructions, as it were, from the bottom of the rock face. The challenge to us as clinicians, and as scientists, was to participate in mindfulness, to experience it from the inside. We committed ourselves to developing a regular mindfulness meditation practice.

Committing to doing something is one thing; doing it is quite another. We experienced many struggles in doing this "simple" thing that we had asked our patients to do. Finding time in a busy schedule, or perhaps getting up 45 minutes earlier than usual, was difficult. There were, we discovered, a wonderful array of excuses on a particular day to take a break from the discipline of daily practice. Then, there was the issue of how much of this we could disclose to professional colleagues (a minor issue, as it turned out; it constantly surprises us how many of our colleagues also do some practice like this and have not told anyone). We remembered what we had heard mindfulness instructors say to their patients: that taking the stress reduction classes is stressful. Now we knew what they meant. Apart from anything else, we found that our respect for our patients rose enormously; perhaps even more for those who struggle and struggle yet still turn up each week for the class.

As time passed, we were able to incorporate the experience with the mindfulness practice into our further reading, into discussions with each other, and with the teachers at the Stress Reduction Clinic in our subsequent visits. Our difficulties in implementing attentional control training had taught us something very important. It had helped us to realize that the approach we had been developing to reduce relapse in depressed patients required revision, and we now felt we could look again to see what these revisions should be. Our perspective about what patients needed to learn in class and in homework had changed radically. We found ourselves more confident that patients already had within themselves the resources they needed to move forward in the way they handled their problems. The issue turned on how best to empower them to do so, and this would require us to change both our theory and practice.

IMPLICATIONS FOR OUR APPROACH: THE NATURE OF DECENTERING

We could now see that our theoretical analysis had taken us only part of the way. We had stressed the importance of the change in relationship to thoughts that cognitive therapy brought about when it protected a person against relapse. This is what we had meant by decentering. But we could now see that our understanding of "decentering" was at once too specific, yet not specific enough.

In the first place, our understanding was too specific, because it referred mainly to thoughts. This was quite understandable, given that our starting point had been an attempt to understand the role of decentering in thought change in cognitive therapy. But the MBSR program was teaching people to explore how they might have a different relationship not only to thoughts but *also* to feelings and bodily sensations.

In the second place, our understanding of "decentering" was not specific enough. Decentering is an ambiguous term: It can be done in a number of ways, and with a number of different attitudes. For example, decentering can be seen as a "stepping away from." But this might mean ignoring a problem and hoping it will go away. Or it might mean trying to dissociate from thoughts or feelings to suppress, repress, or otherwise avoid them. The mode of mind one brings to decentering is critical. The stance of the mindfulness approach is one of *welcoming* and *allowing*. It is invitational. It encourages "opening" to the difficult and adopting an attitude of gentleness to all experience.

Broadening the scope of decentering beyond the realm of thinking brings all experience within this attitude of allowing and welcoming. So long as we focused only on thoughts, we offered participants a restricted view of the means to deal with negative feelings and sensations. Broadening the scope might allow participants to learn how they might deal directly with feelings and body sensations, rather than (as we had planned in attentional control training) dealing with negative feelings by identifying and changing related patterns of negative thought. Extending the application of decentering to feelings and bodily sensations allowed more "ways in" to difficult experiences.

Even when the negative thinking was the predominant feature, this alternative approach allowed participants to handle such negative thoughts by taking, as it were, a "friendly awareness" to the parts of the body affected by the thought–affect cycle. The difficulty of describing these processes in words further emphasizes the importance of understanding them "from the inside," from the perspective of ongoing mindfulness practice.

TEACHING PEOPLE A NEW WAY OF RELATING TO EXPERIENCE

Looking back now, it is understandable, given where we were coming from, that we would see mindfulness as a technique that could fit straightforwardly into a cognitive therapy framework. In our own training, we had been taught that when faced with a difficult clinical problem, we should collaborate with the patient on how best to solve it by seeing what thoughts, interpretations, and assumptions might be causing or exacerbating the problem. We anticipated taking the same approach in developing attentional control training, bolting mindfulness techniques onto this basic therapy framework. However, it became clear from our later visits to the Stress Reduction Clinic that unless we changed the basic structure of our treatment, we would continually revert to dealing with the most difficult problems by searching for more elaborate ways to fix them. Instead, it now appeared to us that the overarching structure of our treatment program needed to change from a mode in which we were therapists to a mode in which we were instructors. What was the difference? As therapists, coming as we did from the cognitive-behavioral tradition, we felt a responsibility to help patients solve their problems, "untie the knots" of their thinking and feeling, and reduce their distress, staying with a problem until it was resolved. By contrast, we saw that the MBSR instructors left responsibility clearly with the patients themselves, and saw their primary role as empowering patients to relate mindfully to their experience on a moment-by-moment basis.

Instructors in MBSR encouraged participants to let go of the idea that problems might, with enough effort, be "fixed." If fixing worked, then fine. But the mindfulness approach was explicit about the danger that such attempts at fixing might merely reinforce people's attitude that their problems were the "enemy," and that once they were eliminated, then everything would be fine. The problem is that this approach may encourage further attempts to solve problems by ruminating on them, and these attempts often keep people trapped in the state from which they are trying to escape. This is something that family therapists have emphasized for years;[69] it is central to Marsha Linehan's concept of self-invalidation,[62] and there is good experimental support for the notion.[70]

Of course, it is understandable that someone who is in distress will want to avoid further suffering. The MBSR approach, however, was that a skillful response would involve, first, recognizing how quickly we react, by jumping in to try to solve the problem. It emphasized letting go of the attempts at problem solving and, instead, purposely standing back to see what it feels like to see the problem through the lens of nonreactivity, and to bring a kindly awareness to the difficulty. The aim was to see the problem and whatever needed to be done clearly, to address the problem in a more skillful way.

This approach ran somewhat counter to the commonly held, but mistaken, view of mindfulness as a way to escape or shut out unwanted thoughts and feelings. The MBSR instructors did not help participants shut off or exit their negative experiences. Instead, they tried to show patients how fighting against unwanted thoughts, feelings, and bodily sensations sometimes created more tension and inner turmoil. With time, some of the tension itself could be reduced. Instead of continuously "feeding" the tension by participating in what their thoughts or feelings demanded, participants stayed close to this mental struggle by finding a calm place from which to observe it.[63]

We could see more clearly why MBSR used body-focused awareness exercises, including a body scan exercise that involved focusing awareness on each part of the body in turn, as well as stretches, mindful walking, and yoga. These were not simply added extras, but a central way in which a person might learn to relate differently to his or her experience. The MBSR approach allows participants to see how negative thoughts and feelings are often expressed through the body. These sensations, too, could be held in awareness and observed, not pushed away. Awareness of the effect of negative thoughts and feelings in the body gave participants another place to stand, another perspective from which to view the situation. This awareness discouraged avoidance of difficult or painful thoughts, feelings, or body sensations. Instead, it suggested a measured and reliable way of "turning toward" and "looking into" these experiences. It also suggested that breathing or a neutral focus in the body could be used as a base or center from which to steady oneself if the work of looking at one's experience became overwhelming. Both of these ideas seemed to have the effect of "leveling the playing field," so that any experience regardless of its valence or importance, was seen as worthy of the person's attention.

Based on what we had seen, we concluded that class members were not just being exposed to a set of skills or techniques to be used at the first sign of stress. They were actually learning *a more general mode of mind that was especially helpful in relating to difficult experiences*. Participants' regular meditation was teaching them to understand the nature of their thoughts, simply as thoughts, and to observe the relationship they had to them. More than that, their meditation also cultivated a new attitude toward all experience, including feelings and body sensations.

MINDFULNESS-BASED COGNITIVE THERAPY

In summary, our deeper understanding of what was actually going on in the MBSR program was directly relevant to the difficulties we had experienced in our initial attempt to use attentional control training. We had first come to MBSR through our belief that decentering and developing a different relationship to negative thinking was the key to cognitive therapy's ability to prevent relapse. We found that decentering was also important in the MBSR program. We then tried to use decentering to "nip in the bud" low-level negative thoughts and feelings. However, for more intense feelings, we had reverted to a conventional cognitive therapy approach, only to find there was just not enough time in the attentional control training group context to use this approach effectively. We saw how the MBSR instructor's "decentered" stance, to even the most intense negative experiences, utilized decentering more widely and deeply than we did. We finally realized why Jon Kabat-Zinn had called his book *Full Catastrophe Living*. He and his colleagues were not helping people avoid the catastrophes in their lives, but teaching them how to embrace them and to live in the midst of them. This new perspective provided us with the springboard we needed to move forward.

Having a springboard is one thing; having the resources to allow you to use it is another. Throughout the period of development we have described, we had been drafting and redrafting applications to two funding bodies, both of which finally approved applications that enabled a multicenter research project to go ahead. One grant was from the United Kingdom's National Health Service's Wales Office of Research and Development for Health and Social Care and the other from the National Institute of Mental Health in Washington, DC. These funding bodies allowed us to build on the work we had done for the MacArthur Foundation, to finalize the manual, and to evaluate our prophylactic intervention. The submissions that they approved reflected their interest in the link between the mindfulness intervention and our theoretical model that pointed to the reactivation, at times of lowered mood, of patterns of persistent thought–affect–body cycles similar in kind to the patterns that occurred during a person's previous depressions. We were clearly saying that for depressive relapse, this was the risk factor that needed to be altered.

We could now write the final draft of the treatment manual, out of our new understanding of how best to capture the decentering that we believed had been a critical factor in cognitive therapy. We would do so in the context of a mindfulness approach that would use awareness of all experience as grist for the mill in preventing future depression. We now had an eight-session program that was closely modeled on MBSR yet retained elements of cognitive therapy. The funding meant that we would finally be in a position to submit our model to a scientific test, in the form of a randomized clinical trial. The results of this trial are reported in Chapter 13. In brief, the participants of the 8-week program were much less likely to become depressed again in the 12 months following their participation. Furthermore, we were surprised to find that the more "chronic" cases benefited more from the program than those with a shorter history of depression. Results showed that those who had suffered more episodes of depression in the past, and therefore had the greatest risk of relapse or recurrence, were helped more by the program than those who had experienced fewer episodes and were thus at less risk.

Following the completion of the trial, we became less sure that the title "attention control training" conveyed the essence of the approach. We had incorporated cognitive therapy principles and practice into a mindfulness framework. It had become mindfulness-based cognitive therapy.

CHAPTER 4

❈

Models in Mind

Before starting out on a journey into new territory, it is important to have as clear a map of the terrain as possible. In earlier chapters, we have described the ups and downs of the project, and how our early theoretical model was shaped and reshaped by the research and clinical findings, and by our experience in exploring the mindfulness approach. We have shown how the earlier maps we had drawn needed to be changed. Having redrawn these maps several times, there is a danger that the situation remains rather unclear, that we have left a map so filled with scribbles and amendments that it might be difficult to see which road is going where. Nowhere yet have we described the overall model on which we settled, the map that would guide our use of the mindfulness approach in preventing depression. In this chapter, therefore, we lay out, as best we can, our understanding of the psychological factors involved in the risk of relapse, and therefore, what it is that mindfulness-based cognitive therapy (MBCT) has to do if it is to help people with their vulnerabilities.

There is an additional, important reason for being very clear about what overall model is guiding treatment. Chapters 6–13 describe the program, session by session. You will see that it includes a range of practices, techniques, and exercises. But we believe the effectiveness of the whole is more than the sum of these parts. Our experience with mindfulness training and, before that, cognitive therapy, has convinced us that the techniques that a therapist or instructor uses are, by themselves, not enough. Rather, it is the way that those procedures are woven together with other aspects of the total treatment context that determines just how much change will occur in persons taking part in the program. The most enduring changes in patients seem to come from shifts at a deeper level than simply acquiring a new "bag of tools" of specific skills and techniques for dealing with particular problematic situations, even though acquisition of those skills might have been the vehicle through which the wider shift occurred.

What, exactly, does this mean? This is not an easy question to answer. The key idea is that patients make radical changes in the underlying views, or mental models, that shape their relationship to negative thoughts and feelings. Such shifts in view often occur as the result of the accumulated effects of repeated learning experiences, framed in a particular way, rather than from general discussions of these ideas or the blind application of techniques. We hope that in the following chapters, as we describe the program, session by session, you will get some sense of how it weaves experiential and conceptual input together to create those shifts, and that the accumulating effects will lead to changes in your own mental models. However, reading about others' experiences is not the same as having those experiences yourself. So, we offer here some conceptual scaffolding that may aid your integration of the material in the following chapters into changes in underlying views in your mind. In doing so, we inevitably repeat some of what we have discussed in Chapters 1–3. The aim here is to draw from that material an integrated model that underlies the MBCT program.

The ultimate aim of the MBCT program is to help individuals make a radical shift in their relationship to the thoughts, feelings, and bodily sensations that contribute to depressive relapse, and to do so through changes in understanding at a deep level. The instructor's own basic understanding and orientation will be one of the most powerful influences affecting this process. Whether the instructor realizes it or not, this understanding colors the way each practice is presented, each interaction is handled. The cumulative effect of such coloring is that, whatever the explicit message of the instructor's words, the more powerful influence, for good or ill, will be the nature of the instructor's basic, implicit understanding. So let us, as best we can, describe the concepts that, we believe, underpin effective use of MBCT.

WHAT'S THE PROBLEM?

One of the great strengths of cognitive therapy is that it provides a way to look at the links between the feelings, thoughts, and behaviors that make up a particular emotional disorder. As well as giving the therapist and client a mental map to make sense of the clinical condition they are working on, this understanding provides guidance as to what needs to be changed to make things better. As a result, both therapist and client can use their energies flexibly and creatively to address problems, rather than being limited to "technique" as a way out of difficulties, by mindless application of a narrow range of fixed procedures.

In the same way, it is really helpful if the instructor in a MBCT program has a working understanding of the processes that maintain depression and, especially, that underlie relapse after recovery— changing these is, of course, the aim of the whole endeavor. Yet, for most, if not all, of the program, participants will probably not actually experience these processes directly. They are not severely depressed at the moment, so their worst moods and thoughts are simply not available to be "put on the workbench," so that they can learn new ways of dealing with them. In this situation, we need an understanding that points to aspects of everyday experiences that share similar underlying mechanisms with the processes that bring about relapse. Once we have that understanding, these aspects of everyday experience can be used as grist for learning in the program. So how are we to understand the processes of relapse, and how are these processes related to everyday experiences?

UNDERSTANDING RELAPSE:
A WORKING MODEL

Relapse involves the reactivation, at times of lowering mood, of patterns of negative thinking similar to the thought patterns that were active during people's previous episodes of depression. Reactivation of these patterns is automatic. It comes about by itself rather than as the result of a deliberate decision by the person. Indeed, the reappearance of these old patterns of thought is often the last thing for which the person would wish. The patterns themselves also seem automatic, in the sense that the mind runs around some very well-worn mental grooves, or ruts, as old mental habits switch in and run off. Again, the thinking here is more a matter of the mind "doing its own thing" than conscious decision and choice.

Although we speak of patterns of negative thinking, in fact, relapse involves the reactivation of a whole, integrated, package of characteristic thoughts, feelings, and physical sensations. These different components of the package interact in ways that reinforce each other through feedback loops that keep regenerating, afresh, the whole constellation of thoughts, feelings, and physical sensations. In this way, an ongoing state of mind is maintained. If left unchecked, this state of mind can lead to the more severe and persistent depression that characterizes relapse.

At the heart of this state of mind is a particular "view" or "model" of depressive experience. Within this view, the self is seen (or, more precisely, felt) as inadequate, worthless and blameworthy, and negative thoughts are seen as accurate reflections of reality. This view, or model, is much more than simply a collection of concepts or ideas about the self and depression. Rather, it represents the distilled essence of many experiences of mind, feelings, and body. This essence is represented at a level deeper than the purely conceptual. If we are to make changes at this deeper level, we need to do more than provide patients with new conceptual information about depression, negative thinking, and relapse. Instead, we need to provide new experiences for the mind and body, over and over again, that will accumulate to create an alternative view.

WHAT KEEPS OLD MENTAL HABITS
IN PLACE?

If relapse involves the reactivation of old mental habits, how was it that the mind picked up these bad habits in the first place, and, more to the point, why should it have kept them when they seem to be so unhelpful? The best answer seems to be that these states of mind are actually motivated to achieve highly desired ends. Perhaps the most salient goal is to prevent or reduce these states of mind themselves. But the strategies used to achieve these ends are actually quite counterproductive. They have exactly the opposite effect to that intended. Take, for example, a person who is still upset for days after a store clerk has been rude or an acquaintance has taken 2 days to return a phone call. He or she may remain upset, not so much because of the original situation, but because his or her mind goes round and round trying to work out why he or she got so upset in the first place. Instead of helping people out of the hole into which they find themselves sinking, worrying away at it (running off these old mental habits) means that people dig themselves deeper into the very hole from which they are trying to escape.

There is a tragic mismatch between the cognitive strategies built into these old mental habits and what is actually required to change such a self-perpetuating state of mind. The old mental habits deceive people into attempting to "think" their way out of their problems. This involves ruminatively dwelling on current emotional states, past negative events, and all the problems that will be created if things don't change. At the heart of this rumination is what we might call a "discrepancy monitor": a process that continually monitors and evaluates the state of the self and the current situation against a model or standard of what is desired, required, expected, or feared. Once this discrepancy monitor is switched on, it will find mismatches between current and desired states. That is its job. Such mismatches may motivate further attempts to reduce these discrepancies, but they also fuel the generation of further undesired negative mood. In this way, attempts to solve problems by endlessly thinking about them can serve merely to keep individuals locked into the state from which they are trying to escape.

If a person has had previous experience with the awfulness of major depression, it is entirely understandable that he or she would be deeply invested in avoiding further depression, and persist in attempts to escape or avoid depression in the face of repeated failure. However, a more skillful response might simply be to abandon those attempts and disengage from the relapse-engendering state of mind. How can this be done?

CHANGING MODES OF MIND

We can think of the mind as an assembly of interacting components. Each of these components receives information arising from the world of the senses or from other components of the mind. Each component processes the information it receives and passes the processed information on to other components. These components then do the same, and pass on more information. We can think of the workings of the mind as a continuous flow and exchange of information among its components. If we could look into the mind, we would notice that, over time, there are certain recurring patterns in the interactions among its components. For a while, one pattern predominates, and then, in response to changes in the external or internal worlds, a shift occurs, so that the same components of mind that previously interacted in one pattern now do so in a different configuration. This interaction then prevails for a longer or shorter time until a further shift occurs, either back to the original pattern of interaction or to yet another configuration. In this way, we could see the activity of the mind as continually shifting, recurring, or evolving patterns of interaction among its components—a little like a car driven through a busy city undergoes a continuous sequence of gear shifts.

If we think of recurring patterns of interaction among mental components as modes of mind, loosely analogous to the gears of a car, then certain aspects of the analogy can help us understand such modes. Just as each gear has a particular use (starting, accelerating, cruising, etc.), so each mode of mind has a characteristic function. In a car, a change of gear can be prompted either automatically (with an automatic transmission, because a device detects when the engine speed reaches certain critical values) or intentionally (with a manual gearshift, because the driver makes a conscious decision to change gear). In the same way, modes of mind can change either automatically (triggered in response to particular kinds of information processing) or intentionally (the individual consciously chooses to rehearse a particular intention or to deploy attention in a particular way). Equally, just as a car cannot be simultaneously in two gears, because both gears require exclusive access to a single engine, so the mind cannot at the same time be in two modes that require exclusive use of the same mental components. Operating in certain modes of mind automatically precludes being in certain other states of mind at the same time.

We can think of the task of mindfulness training as teaching individuals ways to become more aware of their mode of mind ("mental gear") at any moment, and the skills to disengage, if they choose, from unhelpful modes of mind and to engage more helpful modes. We can describe this process as learning how to shift mental gears. In practice, this task often comes down to recognizing two main modes in which the mind operates and learning the skills to move from one to the other. Traditionally, these two modes have been known as "doing" and "being."

"Doing" Mode

The doing mode (we might also have called it the "driven" mode) is triggered when the mind sees that things are other than it would like them to be. Stated more formally, the doing mode is entered when the mind registers discrepancies between an idea of how things are (or of how they are expected to become) and an idea of how things are *wished* to be, or of how things *ought* to be. Such discrepancies do two things: First, they automatically trigger some form of negative feeling; second, they set in motion certain habitual patterns of mind that are designed to reduce the gap between present (or anticipated) state and desired state.

If action can be taken straightaway to reduce the discrepancy, and such action is successful, the mind may exit the doing mode. But what happens when the action to be taken is not obvious, or cannot be implemented immediately? For example, if you are upset because a long-standing relationship has just ended, many potential discrepancies occur between current reality and how you might wish things to be. You may wish for restoration of the relationship, or for the start of another relationship, and you might also wish that you were not so upset. There may be solutions you could find. But what if you begin to feel that you are bound to end up alone, because you conclude that there is some basic failure about you as a person that caused the relationship to fail? This conclusion suggests no ready solution, and the discrepancy remains. The result is that the mind continues to process all the information in "doing" mode, going round and round, dwelling on the discrepancy and rehearsing possible ways to reduce it. This will continue until the discrepancy is reduced or some more urgent task leads to a temporary switch in the topic that the mind processes, only to return to the unresolved discrepancy once the alternative task becomes less of a priority.

What does the doing (driven) mode feel like subjectively? The most common feature is a recurring sense of unsatisfactoriness, caused by the very fact that the mind focuses its processing on the mismatches between how you would like things to be and how they are. It also involves the continuous monitoring and evaluation of progress toward reducing the gap between these two states. Why? Because in those cases where the discrepancies relate to topics about which no immediate action can be taken, the only action that the mind can take is to continue to manipulate its ideas (its representations about how things are and how they are wished to be), in the hope of finding a way to reduce the gap between them. This it will do over and over again. In this situation, because the "currency" with which the mind is working consists of thoughts about current situations, desired situations, explanations for the discrepancies between them, and possible ways to reduce those discrepancies, these thoughts and concepts will be experienced, mentally, as "real" rather than simply as events in the mind. Equally, the mind will not be fully tuned in to the full actuality of present experience. It will be so preoccupied with analyzing the past or the future that the present is given a low priority. In this case, people will only be aware of the present in a very narrow sense: The only interest in it is to monitor success or failure at meeting goals. The broader sense of the present, in what might be called its "full multidimensional splendor," is missed.

In the interest of providing a balanced account, we should point out that conceptual, discrepancy-based, problem solving, if applied intentionally and knowingly to problems for which it is appropriate, is, of course, one of the most impressive attributes of the human mind. The very success of this approach, when used in this way, is the understandable reason such strategies become incorporated into the doing mode in the first place. The problem is that, in the doing mode, processing is usually not intentional, conscious, and planned; rather, it begins and is maintained relatively automatically, as a mental habit "in the back of the mind." In this situation, the mind may well drive itself round in circles or switch from one unresolved discrepancy to another, without ever reaching resolution. This is likely to be particularly true in relation to the lifelong goals, such as being more happy or less unhappy, that many of us carry around, and that are processed in the background as the mind's default priority, when the mind is not otherwise engaged.

The negative thought patterns reactivated at times of potential relapse are aspects of a state of mind that, itself, is a variant of the basic "doing" mode. As happens at other times when we are upset, negative mood may trigger the doing mode of mind. People notice that they feel bad; they want to feel better. There is a mismatch between the actual and the desired state of affairs. The doing mode is automatically switched on. Unfortunately, as we saw with relapse-related processing, the doing mode is often not the most skillful response to unwanted emotion and, in vulnerable individuals, may actually serve to enhance and maintain the unwanted emotion rather than reduce it. The same is true of other forms of emotional discomfort.

The importance of this, from our point of view, is that the parallels between the manifestations of the doing/driven mode in relapse-related processing and in more everyday emotional experience mean that we can use such experience as a training ground on which to learn skills to recognize and disengage from this mode. We return shortly to a discussion of how this might be done. For the moment, let us consider an alternative cognitive mode, that of "being."

"Being" Mode

The full richness of the mode of "being" is not easily conveyed in words—its flavor is best appreciated directly, experientially. In many ways, it is the opposite of the doing mode. Recall that the doing/driven mode is goal-oriented, motivated to reduce the gap between how things are and how we would like them to be; our attention is devoted to the narrow focus on discrepancies between desired and actual states. By contrast, the being mode is not motivated to achieve particular goals. This has two implications. First, there is no need for constant monitoring and evaluation of "how am I doing in meeting my goals?" Second, there is no need to emphasize discrepancy-based processing. Instead, the focus of the being mode is "accepting" and "allowing" what is, without any immediate pressure to change it.

Such "allowing" reflects the fact that, in the absence of a goal or standard to be reached, there is no need to evaluate experience in order to reduce discrepancies between actual and desired states. Instead of narrowly focusing on the present, cursorily processed in terms of its standing with respect to goal achievement, the being mode experience in any moment can be processed in its full depth, width, and richness.

Equally, doing and being differ in their time focus. In doing, it is often necessary to compute the future consequences of goal-related action, anticipate the consequences of goal achievement, or rehearse memories of past problematic or goal-related situations as a way to facilitate current goal achievement. As a result, in doing mode, the mind often travels forward to the future or back to the past, and the experience is one of not actually being "here" in the present much of the time. By contrast, in being mode, the mind has "nothing to do, nowhere to go" and so processing can be dedicated exclusively to the processing of moment-by-moment experience, allowing the individual to be fully present and aware of whatever is. Whereas doing mode involves thinking *about* the present, the future, and the past, relating to each of these through a veil of concepts, being mode is characterized by direct, immediate, intimate experience of the present.

The being mode involves a shift in relation to thoughts and feelings. Conceptual thought is a core vehicle through which the mind seeks to achieve the goals to which the doing mode of mind is dedicated. Accordingly, as we have seen, thought is accorded the status of a valid reflection of reality and closely linked to action. Within the doing mode, feelings are primarily evaluated as "good things" or "bad things" and the mind sets up goals to make sure that they, respectively, continue or cease. Again, making feelings into goal-related objects in this way effectively crystallizes them into "things" that have an independent and enduring reality.

By contrast, in being mode, the relation to thoughts and feelings is much the same as to sounds or other aspects of moment-by-moment experience; these are simply passing events in the mind that arise, become objects of awareness, and then pass away. You will recognize here the "decentered" perspective to which we attached such importance in our analysis of the way that cognitive therapy has its effects. In the being mode, the shift in relation to thoughts and feelings involves a further disconnection of thought and feeling from goal-related action. Feelings do not immediately trigger automatic sequences of action in the mind or body to hang on to pleasant feelings and get rid of unpleasant feelings. This, necessarily, involves a greater ability to tolerate uncomfortable emotional states without immediately triggering habitual patterns of mental or physical action in the attempt to escape or ameliorate those states. Equally, thoughts such as "do this, do that" do not necessarily automatically link to related actions, but can be related to simply as events in the mind.

Finally, being mode is characterized by a sense of freedom, freshness, and unfolding of experience in new ways. It is responsive to the richness and complexity of the unique patterns that each moment presents. In doing mode, by contrast, the multidimensional nature of experience is reduced primarily to a unidimensional analysis of its standing in relation to a goal state. Discrepancies between actual and goal states then trigger fairly well-worn, automatic habits of mind that have been used in many other instances of discrepancy-related processing. As we have seen, for certain goals, such as reducing discrepancy-based emotion, these habits can backfire and lead to perpetuation, rather than cessation, of unwanted mind states.

Before drawing out the implications of the distinction between doing and being modes for MBCT, it is important that we be very clear on one point. We do not mean to imply that being mode is a special state in which all activity has to stop. Doing or being are modes of mind, that can both accompany any activity or lack of activity. Recall that doing mode can also, for most purposes, be renamed the "driven mode" and it may become clearer. For example, it is possible to try to meditate with so much focus on getting to a deeply relaxed state that if anything interrupts it one feels angry and frustrated. That would be meditating in a doing rather than a being mode, because the meditation is "driven" by the desire to relax. Or take another example: It is your turn to do the dishes and there is no way out of it. No one is going to rescue you from this chore. If you do the dishes with the aim of finishing them as quickly as possible to get on to the next activity and are then interrupted, there will be frustration, since your goal has been thwarted. But if you accept that the dishes have to be done and approach the activity in being mode, then the activity exists for its own sake in its own time. An interruption is simply treated as something that presents a choice about what to do at that moment, rather than as a source of frustration.

THE CORE SKILL

The core skill that the MBCT program aims to teach is the ability, at times of potential relapse, to recognize and disengage from mind states characterized by self-perpetuating patterns of ruminative, negative thought. Such patterns, if left unchecked, are likely to produce a downward spiraling of mood, and, eventually, the onset of relapse. In order to do this, participants have to learn how to disengage from one mode of mind and enter another, incompatible, mode of mind that will allow them to process depression-related information in ways that are less likely to provoke relapse. This involves moving from a focus on content to a focus on process, away from cognitive therapy's emphasis on changing the content of negative thinking, toward attending to the way all experience is processed.

The basic tool to effect this change of mental modes, or shift of mental gears, is the intentional use of attention and awareness in particular ways. By choosing what we are going to attend to, and how we are going to attend to it, we place our hand on the lever that enables us to change mental gears.

How do participants in the program learn to do this when, in recovery, the mind states that provoke relapse do not occur very often and are therefore not available for learning? As we have already noted, relapse-related mind states are actually particular examples of the much more general doing/driven mode of mind. In our culture, this doing/driven mode of mind is extremely prevalent and participants will almost certainly engage it as their "default" mode of mind in many situations. This means that the doing mode occurs again and again during the program and may become especially apparent during the exercises, practices, and interactions that take place in the sessions themselves and in the homework. In the sessions, operation of this mode of mind in participants occurs not only under their own noses but also under the nose of the instructor. In this way, with sufficient skill on the part of the instructor, much of the content of the program, both planned and unplanned, can be used as opportunities to recognize and disengage from doing mode. It is, of course, even more helpful if participants can have opportunities to do this work in relation to unpleasant emotional states in general, and to depression in particular. For this reason, the instructor has a very real basis for welcoming the occurrence of such states as "grist for the mill" and ideal opportunities for teaching the core skills at the heart of the program.

When can participants find opportunities to cultivate being mode? In principle, this mode of mind can be practiced in all situations. In practice, the tendency to enter doing mode is so pervasive (especially when one is learning a new skill such as how to "be"!) that very simple learning situations have to be set up, and the instructor has to embody being mode more or less constantly in those situations in order to facilitate entry into this mode of mind.

The doing mode has a strong tendency to keep itself going and to reassert itself once the mind has switched to another mode of processing. It is particularly important, therefore, that the mode to which the mind switches after disengaging from doing mode be mutually incompatible and inconsistent with doing mode, just as it is not possible to be in forward and reverse gears in a car at one and the same time. Being mode is an ideal candidate for such an initial, alternative mode into which to switch from doing mode. Once that initial switch has been made, it may be appropriate for patients to learn how to enter, intentionally, some other mode, for example, one that will facilitate skillful, planned action to alleviate any persisting depressed mood.

In the end, we need to balance both of these modes in our lives. Whether it is because the culture we live in exalts doing, or because doing mode is often propelled by automatic, well-worn routines, it can easily crowd out other ways of being with one's experience. We can learn to switch out of automatic pilot by bringing our awareness to the present moment. When we do this, we start to see that we have a choice, and this is often the first step in taking care of ourselves differently in the face of sad moods.

MINDFULNESS AS CORE SKILL

Mindfulness has been described as "paying attention in a particular way: on purpose, in the present moment, and nonjudgmentally" (p. 4).[63] As such, mindfulness fits remarkably well the requirements that our analysis has identified as a core skill to be learned in a relapse prevention program. Awareness of the patterns of thought, feelings, and bodily sensations that characterize relapse-related mind states (and the doing mode of mind more generally) is an essential first step in recognizing the need for corrective action. Intentionally (on purpose) changing the focus and style of attention is the "mental gear lever" by which processing can be switched from one cognitive mode to another. And the nonjudgmental, present moment, focus of mindfulness indicates that it is indeed very closely related to the being mode of mind. In other words, mindfulness provides both the means to change mental gears when disengaging from dysfunctional, "doing-related" mind states, and an alternative mental gear, or incompatible mode of mind, into which to switch.

THE STRUCTURE
OF THE MINDFULNESS-BASED
COGNITIVE THERAPY PROGRAM

In Part II, we describe in detail, session by session, the MBCT program. Immersed in the detail of each session, it is easy to lose sight of the overall aim and structure of the program. It may therefore be helpful to remember that the aim of early sessions is to teach participants to recognize doing mode in its many manifestations and to begin the cultivation of being mode by intensive, formal mindfulness practice. You will see this theme repeated quite a lot as the sessions unfold. Such repetition is there to remind participants again and again of the core themes, for practice provides many opportunities to recognize that being mode is no longer present, to disengage from the prevailing mode, and to return to mindful being mode. As mindfulness skills develop, training focuses more specifically on recognizing when, in everyday life, negative emotions and reactions trigger doing mode, and on learning how to disengage from that mode, enter being mode, and, how, if necessary, to simply *be with* difficult and uncomfortable emotions. Subsequently, the simple skill of disengagement from emotion-related modes of mind is supplemented by additional coping strategies that provide patients with a range of options for responding more skillfully to negative emotion. Finally, the skills taught are integrated around the ultimate aim of the program: staying well and preventing future relapse.

PART II

⌘

Mindfulness-Based Cognitive Therapy

CHAPTER 5

☒

The Eight-Session Program

HOW AND WHY

The chapters that follow this one aim to give a detailed sense of mindfulness-based cognitive therapy (MBCT), session by session. Those who are primarily interested in getting the flavor of MBCT may, after reading this introduction, proceed straight to Chapter 6, where we begin to describe Session 1. The present chapter is intended for those who contemplate the possibility of actually doing MBCT. Here, we focus in some detail on the "how and why" of running sessions within this approach. Some may find it helpful to return to this section after reading the description of the eight-session program. Others may find this chapter a useful opportunity to ground their perception of MBCT in concrete detail, before going on to the more narrative description that follows.

For those interested in pursuing this approach further, we have provided more practical details both in this introduction and by including the handouts that we gave, section by section, to participants after each session (including details of the homework following that session). We have included a short chapter in Part III, "Going Further" (Chapter 15) with addresses, websites, and other resources that we hope will be helpful.

In describing each session, we aim to do a number of things: to say what we intended each session to include, and describe what we observed; to let participants themselves speak about their discoveries with the practice; to speak frankly about where we, as teachers, found things difficult, and how we attempted to understand what was going on when such difficulties arose. The style is somewhat different than that we have used up until now. There are poems, parables, and stories, and the world of the psychology textbook seems even further away. There are many repetitions: The stream of argument sometimes seems to loop back on itself (many times), and it may feel like the stream will never reach the river, nor the river the sea. Our hope is that, gradually, a more complete picture will emerge from the individual parts, just as, for participants in the program, the same message in the context of different sessions made sense to them the second or third time they heard it, when it had not even been noticed before.

PRACTICAL ISSUES

Working with Recovered Depressed Patients

There are a number of constraints in working with people who have had such serious episodes of depression. First, because they may have overcome their episodes of depression with the help of antidepressants, they may have a "biological" model of their illness. Such a model is perfectly understandable given their experience, and any psychosocial approach needs to take account of it. With this in mind, we suggest taking time during initial assessment interviews (see later) to discuss how both biological and psychosocial factors may play a role in the onset, maintenance, and recurrence of depression.

A second constraint in working with recovered patients is that, in remission, symptoms of depression are, by definition, "low level." Previous psychological treatments developed for depression assume that clients experience relatively "loud" phenomena—persistent low mood, negative thoughts and images, severe biases in memory and judgment, inability to experience pleasure and inactivity, and suicidal thoughts and impulses. An important aim of the mindfulness-based approach is therefore to teach clients to be more aware of even small changes in their mood. Since the symptoms are not "loud," clients are taught to listen for the whisper.

A third constraint is that recurrence, when it comes, will not occur until, on average, a year has passed. Teaching clients *about* such recurrence by simply extending their *knowledge* of how to prevent relapse is unlikely to affect an event that is so far in the future. The aim must therefore be to teach *procedures and skills*. MBCT emphasizes daily practice during the active phase of the program, in the expectation that participants will learn skills they cannot easily forget, precisely because they have learned a new way of being in their lives. As part of the research trial described in Chapter 13, we also scheduled four follow-up meetings in the year following the 8-week program. Such follow-up may not be suitable in all settings, but some type of continuing contact will always be valuable. At the Center for Mindfulness at UMass, all past patients are invited each year to one of six regular, all-day retreats that occur between Sessions 6 and 7 as part of MBSR. In this way, "graduates" from previous classes have at least six chances a year to meet and practice with current participants in the MBSR program. In North Wales, all graduates from both research classes and more recent MBSR classes may attend monthly continuation classes. The format for these "graduate classes" is similar to the eight MBCT classes, starting with practice (choosing body scan, sitting meditations, or yoga stretches), then letting the dialogue flow, interwoven with stories or poetry, or further practice. Whatever means are chosen, offering some chance for participants to reconnect with the formal practice in a class setting is important.

Having Your Own Practice

In addition to recognized training in counseling or psychotherapy, or as a mental health professional, with some training in cognitive therapy and in running groups, it is important that instructors have firsthand, ongoing experience of mindfulness practice. Why is this so? First, it is inevitable that some patients will experience difficulties with the practice that the instructor will not be able to answer with "intellectual" knowledge alone. A swimming analogy may help to illustrate the point. A swimming instructor is not someone who knows the physics of how solids behave in liquids, but he or she knows how to swim. It is not just an issue of credibility and competence, but of teachers' ability to embody "from the inside" the attitudes they invite participants to cultivate and adopt. When we started this work, we believed that it was unreasonable to expect all instructors to have experienced such mindfulness practice, or even to have practiced before. We have changed our minds about this.

Our own conclusion, after seeing for ourselves the difference between using MBCT with and without personal experience of using mindfulness practice, is that it is unwise for instructors to embark on teaching this material before they have extensive personal experience with its use. We therefore recommend that, as a minimum, prospective instructors experience using mindfulness in their own daily lives before they embark on teaching it to clients.

For those new to this approach, we give some pointers for how to go about this in Chapter 15, "Going Further."

Planning and Preparation for Sessions

Each session contains a large amount of work to be done: There are always the relevant handouts to distribute; tapes and reading material; the inevitable setting up of the room before each session, perhaps writing key issues on the blackboard and positioning the chairs. In other words, each session needs *planning*. But we found (often to our disadvantage, when we had not left sufficient time for it) that each session also needed *preparation*; that is, we needed to prepare ourselves. When looking at the videotapes of our sessions after the research was over, we could easily identify the times when we had just rushed in from another meeting versus those when we had prepared ourselves by taking the time for things to settle. With this in mind, we recommend that you prepare yourself for each session, so that you approach each class with not only practical arrangements running smoothly but also being able to embody the balance of openness and "groundedness" that participants are invited to experience for themselves. But there is another factor: A sense of preparation that comes from your ongoing mindfulness practice. This will allow you some degree of flexibility of approach in the classes: to stay in the moment and, if necessary, let go of the plan you have made, drawing on other components of the MBCT program to respond to what is most cogent in the participants' experience.

Such talk of careful preparation may give an impression that the aim is to "succeed." Our final word should therefore be one of caution. At the outset, doing this work may create more stress! Just finding 45 minutes a day for yourself to listen to a tape may demand many lifestyle changes. Both instructors and participants may understandably expect some gain from such sacrifice. But the more such expectation of change is uppermost in your mind, the more elusive it may become. As best you can, therefore, suspend judgment and invite participants to do the same. Emphasize the empirical approach. To borrow from the first formal practice used in the program, "Don't try too hard—whatever comes up accept it, for that is what you are feeling right now."

OVERVIEW OF MINDFULNESS-BASED COGNITIVE THERAPY

The Initial Assessment Interview

This initial assessment interview, which lasts around 1 hour, is conducted with each prospective participant and is based on the initial material sent to participants before they attend (see Handout 5.1). This material explains some aspects of depression and the program, and can be used as a starting point for dialogue between instructor and participant. The aim of the initial interview is as follows:

1. To learn about the factors that for each participant have been associated with the onset and maintenance of depression.
2. To explain something of the background of MBCT and explore with each participant how it might help him or her.
3. To emphasize that MBCT will involve some hard work, and a need for patience and persistence in that work, over the course of the 8 weeks.
4. To determine whether the person is likely to benefit at this time. At the Stress Reduction Clinic at UMass, instructors will not take persons into the program if (a) they are actively

suicidal *and* have no other form of counseling support (they are admitted to MBSR if they have other such support); (b) they are currently abusing drugs or alcohol.

The Classes

An outline *theme and curriculum* for each of the eight classes is reproduced at or near the beginning of each session, and the *participant handouts* that we used in our research on MBCT are reproduced at the end of each session. Follow-up classes may be arranged to suit the circumstances. In our research, we arranged for four follow-up classes during the year following the 8-week program (but see earlier discussion).

Class Size

Class size depends on the facilities available. Jon Kabat-Zinn and his colleagues work with classes of 30 or larger, but embedding cognitive therapy techniques in MBCT probably requires smaller classes. We had classes of up to 12 in our research, but MBSR instructors have pointed out that a smaller class can be more problematic because it too easily reverts to a "therapy" rather than a "class" mode.

Core Aims

- To help people who have suffered from depression in the past to learn skills to help prevent depression coming back.
- To become more aware of bodily sensations, feelings, and thoughts, from moment to moment.
- To help participants develop a different way of relating to sensations, thoughts, and feelings—specifically, mindful acceptance and acknowledgment of unwanted feelings and thoughts, rather than habitual, automatic, preprogrammed routines that tend to perpetuate difficulties.
- To help participants be able to choose the most skillful response to any unpleasant thoughts, feelings, or situations that they meet.

The Structure

MBCT prioritizes learning how to pay attention, on purpose, in each moment, and without judgment. Learning to pay attention is the focus of *Sessions 1–4*. First, participants become aware of how little attention is usually paid to daily life. They are taught to become aware of how quickly the mind shifts from one topic to another. Second, they learn how, having noticed that the mind is wandering, to bring it back to a single focus. This is taught, first, with reference to parts of the body and, second, with reference to breathing. Third, the participants learn to become aware of how this mind wandering can allow negative thoughts and feelings to occur.

Only when a person has become aware of these aspects is he or she likely to use MBCT to be vigilant for mood shifts, and then move on to handle them (at the time) or deal with them later. Handling mood shifts now or dealing with them later involves the second phase of MBCT and is dealt with in *Sessions 5–8*. Whenever a negative thought or feeling arises, the instructions emphasize allowing it to simply be there, before taking steps to respond skillfully by using specific strategies. How is this done? Participants learn how to become fully aware of the thought or feeling, and then, having acknowledged it, to move their attention to their breathing for a minute or two before expanding attention to the body as a whole. Taking such a *breathing space* may itself be sufficient to handle difficulties in the moment, to dissolve the unpleasant thought or feeling. In any event, it is seen as the essential first step in dealing with difficulties. Thereafter, participants may choose how best to respond. They may choose to deal with it directly (then or later), by seeing it as simply a thought or feeling and watching it as it passes. Or they may choose to deal with it by noting the part of the body it affects, and bringing awareness to that part of the body, using the breath to open and soften to the sensation rather than tighten and brace around it. Or they may choose to deal with difficulty by taking action specifically chosen for its ability in the past to bring some pleasure or sense of mastery. Because of the large variety of contexts in which the breathing space will be used, it may be important to emphasize its *flexibility*. It will not always be possible for participants to close their eyes and take exactly 3 minutes, but pausing to acknowledge what is going on, to gather themselves by going to the breath before expanding the focus of attention to sense the wider perspective of the here and now is the important first step.

Finally, participants are encouraged to become more aware of their own unique warning signs of impending depression, and to develop specific action plans for when this might occur. We came to believe that MBCT should combine both the generic themes of mindfulness approaches in general and help in dealing with the specific problems that depression poses. But all the time, in the background, was the overall theme of changing the relationship with what was most difficult.

Differences in Participants' Approach to the Classes

Participants' different past experiences account for their very different ways of approaching the classes. Some know a great deal of what the classes will be about; many know nothing and are very scared of what they may be asked to talk about or do. We take time at the start of the first class not only to emphasize confidentiality but also to say that, after they have introduced themselves to the group, participants need feel no pressure at all to say anything during the classes. We also talk at that point about the skill of really *listening* to what another person is saying. By contrast, quite often we spend time, while someone else is talking, working out how we can best help participants, or determining what we are going to say next. Learning to pay attention means learning to be really attentive to what others are saying, while they are saying it. Those who choose to say little may nevertheless contribute much to the class by their very presence (after all, they are *there*), as well as by using their gift of listening.

We found that the way we led the formal practice set the scene for the rest of each class. Some of the instructions we gave ourselves to help us embody the approach are as follows:

• Use the present participle when describing actions you would like participants to take. For example, ". . . just noticing whether your mind has wandered . . . " or ". . . bringing your attention back to the breath . . . " (rather than "Notice whether . . . " or "Bring your attention back . . . ").

• Start the meditation by asking people to spend a few moments being aware of their posture. It is recommended that the back be erect, but not stiff. If someone is sitting on a chair, then it is important to sit partly forward in the seat, so that the back is not supported by the chair frame. Of course, if the person has a bad back or back pain then some type of support for the back may be necessary. Encourage participants to check the alignment of their back, neck, and head. Intentionally creating a posture that embodies dignity, stability, and alertness allows us to bring these qualities to the sitting itself.

• Deliver the instructions for the meditation in a matter-of-fact way. Note that this is not a relaxation exercise, so there is no need to adopt a special tone or deepen the voice to relax the participants. Do not *read* verbatim instructions. Do not *read* instructions out loud at all.

• When giving encouragement, use the phrase "as best you can" rather than using the word "try." For example, ". . . as best you can, bringing your awareness to settle on the breath" rather than "try to bring your awareness to the breath. . . . "

• Do the practice with the class. This means that you are guiding out of your own moment-to-moment experience during the guided meditations.

• Allow for spaces and stretches of silence between your instructions. Give participants the space to "do" the practice for themselves.

GUIDING PRACTICE

We found that the best timing for reflection on class practice is immediately following it. We adopted the practice of never moving on to the next part of the session without giving people an opportunity to respond to and comment on their experience of the practice that has just ended. We came to see this dialogue within the classes as having two stages. First, we asked people to describe their actual experience during the practice. What sensations, thoughts, and feelings came up, and what did people notice about them? Second, we asked whether anyone had any *comments* on their experiences.

Welcoming and staying attentive to what is offered empowers

other group members and contributes to the sense that what they have experienced is legitimate. The instructor's curiosity about participants' experience can invite participants themselves to become curious about their own experience. During the dialogue that took place, therefore, we found it was important to keep close to (and bring the focus back to) participants' actual experience.

The links that class members can see between their own experiences and those of others are very important. We encouraged participants to discuss any difficulties or objections they had. If one person was thinking about them, then somebody else was likely to be thinking about them too.

Finally, bear in mind that different people may find different aspects of MBCT helpful. For some, it may provide useful distraction techniques when they have low mood. It may help others sleep more restfully. For still others, dissolving the troubling thoughts and images in the breathing exercise may change the nature of the experience itself. The aspect of MBCT that is most helpful for each person cannot be prejudged at the outset. Think of your instructor role as planting seeds. You do not know how long they will take to germinate, and, in a real sense, that is not under your control. As best you can, cultivate instead an openness, a sense of discovery. It is with this sense of curiosity and exploration that we move now to draw together the core themes of MBCT.

THE CORE THEMES OF MINDFULNESS-BASED COGNITIVE THERAPY

In this section, we sum up, as precisely as we can, what we believe are the central themes of this approach to depression.

Exploring How Best to Prevent the Establishment and Consolidation of Patterns of Negative Thinking

Everything is in the service of preventing the consolidation of self-perpetuating patterns of negative thinking that may escalate negative mood states to depressive relapse. It is not the aim to keep negative mind states out of mind altogether, but rather to prevent their establishment when they occur.

What Drives the Old Habits of Thinking?

The patterns of negative thinking are based on old, well-practiced, automatic cognitive routines (often ruminative). They are motivated (ineffectively) by the goal of escaping/avoiding depression or problematic life situations. These unhelpful routines persist because the person remains in a cognitive mode characterized by a number of features:

1. "Automatic pilot"
2. Driven by an overriding wish to get rid of the negative mood, and a strong attachment to the goal of feeling happy
3. Constant monitoring/comparison of current state and desired state
4. Reliance on "verbal" problem-solving techniques

What Is the Core Skill?

The *core skill* to be learned is how to exit (step out of) and stay out of these self-perpetuating cognitive routines. The bottom line is *be mindful (aware), let go*. Letting go means relinquishing involvement in these routines, freeing oneself of the attachment/aversion driving the thinking patterns—*it is the continued attempts to escape or avoid unhappiness, or to achieve happiness that keep the negative cycles turning. The aim of the program is freedom*, not happiness, relaxation, and so on, although these may well be welcome by-products.

Experiential Learning

The required *skills/knowledge* can only be acquired through direct experience. Intellectual knowledge may be helpful (it may also get in the way by setting expectations, goals to be attained, etc.) but, by itself, it is wholly inadequate. Acquisition of the skills requires repeated experiences (perhaps many thousands). Getting enough experience can only be achieved if (1) participants accept the responsibility for the 99.9% of learning that will have to occur outside sessions; (2) all experience is grist for the mill—using awareness/letting go of even quite neutral and apparently harmless automatic thoughts/feelings/body sensations to build up skills to deal with depression-related patterns.

Empowerment

Empowerment of participants is absolutely essential if they are to get the required amount of experience in using mindfulness. In the service of empowerment, learning should be based, whenever possible, on participants' own experience rather than lectures from the instructor, and should embody the assumption that participants are the "experts" on themselves, with a fund of relevant experience and skills already:

- Always ask for feedback immediately after any practice or other exercises in session, and from all homework. This feedback should be the main vehicle for teaching.
- Use open-ended questions and encourage the expression of doubts, difficulties, and reservations.
- Underline the essential teaching point that is implicit or explicit in the feedback given by participants. Be concrete and specific in feedback and instructions.
- Keep track, from homework records, whether homework is actually occurring and hone in on nonadherence.
- Encourage a clear intentionality (not goal orientation) in participants. Help them relate the practice to a personally valued vision.
- Keep a balance between instructions to "let go" of expectations (which can be demotivating if overemphasized) and the willingness to believe that important changes may occur as a result of doing the mindfulness practice.
- Encourage curiosity as the mode of investigating experience, even when such experience appears boring or negative.

What Is to Be Learned?

- *Concentration.* The ability to deploy and maintain attention on a particular focus is central to all other aspects of MBCT. This involves sustained, quality attention that is gathered and focused rather than dispersed and fragmented.

- *Awareness/mindfulness of thoughts, emotions/feelings, bodily sensations.* This is important because we can't intentionally let go of unhelpful patterns unless we are aware of them; because awareness itself removes processing resources that are required for the self-perpetuation of unhelpful patterns, and because awareness of difficulties (particularly in the body) involves bringing our "best mind" to bear in ways that may allow the process to unfold more creatively.

- *Being in the moment.* Instructors can support a moment-by-moment mode by not "trailering," that is, not giving instructions in advance of the time when participants actually need to act on them.

- *Decentering.* This is taught as a way of becoming really aware of thoughts, feelings, and body sensations.

- *Acceptance/nonaversion, nonattachment, kindly awareness.* The motivation fueling the automatic cognitive habits is some form of aversion or desire. For this reason, "acceptance of what is" undercuts the power driving these habits. Acceptance and awareness also allow us to see the "bad thing" or "good thing" in a clearer, wider perspective, so we are better able to respond to the totality of a situation rather than to let just one fragment of it instantly "press our buttons."

- *Letting go.* This is a key skill both in preventing oneself getting into and in stepping out of unhelpful cycles. It is a very important part of both the body scan and mindfulness of breath, and one of the key reasons why the very thing people find most difficult (mind wandering) may be one of the most useful; that is, when people are practicing, and their minds repeatedly wander from the breath or the body, then detecting the wandering, and returning, is probably more important than staying on the breath/body 100% of the time. The outbreath is the natural vehicle used in letting go.

- *"Being" rather than "doing," non-goal attainment, no special state (of relaxation, happiness, peace, etc.) to be achieved.* All the unhelpful patterns are variants of the "doing/driven" mode—concerned with achieving defined end points and monitoring current state against expected, desired, or "should" states. Getting the taste for "being" mode, and being able to enter this at will, provides a powerful alternative route when depression-creating "doing" routines are assembling themselves. The practices, and the instructor's own presence and way of being, provide powerful opportunities for direct "tasting" of this mode—hence the importance of the instructor embodying the qualities being developed to whatever degree possible, and, after Session 1, starting each session with a period of practice. Appropriate pacing and punctuation of the session, and having a single focus at any one time, facilitate this mode.

• *Bringing awareness to the manifestation of a problem in the body.* As well as providing cues to the presence of aversion, stress, and so on, bringing awareness to the bodily manifestation of a problem provides a way to withdraw processing resources from the automatic, unhelpful (goal-oriented) routines, while still keeping the problem "in process" (so as not to reinforce aversion). It allows awareness, as a marker of another mode of processing, to get on with the job and let events unfold, undisturbed by the type of thinking that seeks to resolve discrepancies, strive for goals, or solve problems.

CONCLUDING REMARKS

Many psychologists, counselors, and other mental health workers are drawn to their profession by the wish to help people. Such help can take many forms. Most therapies are quite reasonably founded on the principle of getting as clear a view as possible of what has gone wrong in the past and what is going wrong in the present, then helping the person find the resources to cope better. They are based on the idea that assessing and then removing problems is the aim. At best, these attempts empower persons to manage their lives more successfully, and many people have been helped by a number of such treatments.

Our analysis suggests that this will bring temporary relief only, unless people are able to use that respite to find ways of enhancing their own well-being, taking care of themselves, and relating to their problems in a different way. Both the research data and our clinical experience suggest to us that only when people learn to take a different stance in relation to the "battleground" of their thoughts and feelings will they be able in the future to recognize difficult situations early and deal with them skillfully. Taking this different stance involves sampling a different mode of mind from that which we normally inhabit, and which much therapy also inhabits. It involves replacing the old mode of fixing and repairing problems with a new mode of allowing things to be just as they are, in order to see more clearly how best to respond. The eight sessions described in the next few chapters aim to bring about this different way of relating to experience.

PLEASE READ THIS BEFORE WE MEET.

DEPRESSION

Depression is a very common problem. Twenty percent of adults become severely depressed at some point in their lives. Depression involves both biological changes in the way the brain works and psychological changes—the way we think and feel. Because of this, it is often useful to combine medical treatments for treating depression (which act on the brain) with psychological approaches (which teach new ways to deal with thoughts and feelings).

TREATMENT OF DEPRESSION

When you have been depressed in the past your doctor may have prescribed antidepressants. These work through their effects on the chemical messengers in your brain. In depression, these chemical messengers have often become run down, lowering mood and energy levels, and disturbing sleep and appetite. Correcting these brain chemicals may have taken time, but most people experience improvements in 6 to 8 weeks.

Although antidepressants generally work well in reducing depression, they are not a permanent cure—their effects continue only so long as you keep taking the pills. Your doctor could continue to prescribe antidepressants for months, or even years, since this is now the recommended way to use antidepressants if further depression is to be prevented by this means.

However, many people prefer to use other ways to prevent further depression. This is the purpose of the classes you will be attending.

(cont.)

PREVENTION OF MORE DEPRESSION

Whatever caused your depression in the first place, the experience of depression itself has a number of aftereffects. One of these is a likelihood that you will become depressed again. The purpose of these classes is to improve your chance of preventing further depression. In the classes, you will learn skills to help you handle your thoughts and feelings differently.

Since many people have had depression and are at risk for further depression, you will learn these skills in a class with up to a dozen other people who have also been depressed and treated with antidepressants. In eight 2-hour sessions, the class will meet to learn new ways of dealing with what goes on in our minds, and to share and review experiences with other class members.

After the eight weekly sessions are over, the class will meet again four times over the following few months for reunions and to see how things are progressing.

HOMEWORK: THE IMPORTANCE OF PRACTICE

Together, we will be working to change patterns of mind that often have been around for a long time. These patterns may have become a habit. We can only expect to succeed in making changes if we put time and effort into learning skills.

This approach depends entirely on your willingness to do homework between class meetings. This homework will take at least an hour a day, 6 days a week, for 8 weeks, and involves tasks such as listening to tapes, performing brief exercises, and so on. We appreciate that it is often very difficult to carve out that amount of time for something new in lives that are already very busy and crowded. However, the commitment to spend time on homework is an essential part of the class; if you do not feel able to make that commitment, it would be best not to start the classes.

FACING DIFFICULTIES

The classes and the homework assignments can teach you how to be more fully aware and present in each moment of life. The good news is that this makes life more interesting, vivid, and fulfilling. On the other hand, this means facing what is present, even when it is unpleasant and difficult. In practice, you will find that turning to face and acknowledge difficulties is the most effective way, in the long run, to reduce unhappiness. It is also central to preventing further depression. Seeing unpleasant feelings, thoughts, or experiences clearly, as they arise, means that you will be in much better shape to "nip them in the bud," before they progress to more intense or persistent depressions.

(cont.)

In the classes, you will learn gentle ways to face difficulties, and will be supported by the instructor and the other class members.

PATIENCE AND PERSISTENCE

Because we will be working to change well-established habits of mind, you will be putting in a lot of time and effort. The effects of this effort may only become apparent later. In many ways, it is much like gardening—we have to prepare the ground, plant the seeds, ensure that they are adequately watered and nourished, and then wait patiently for results.

You may be familiar with this pattern from your treatment with antidepressants: Often there is little beneficial effect until you have been taking the medication for some time. Yet improvement in your depression depended on your continuing to take the antidepressant even when you felt no immediate benefit.

In the same way, we ask you to approach the classes and homework with a spirit of patience and persistence, committing yourself to put time and effort into what will be asked of you, while accepting, with patience, that the fruits of your efforts may not show straight away.

THE INITIAL INDIVIDUAL MEETING

Your initial individual meeting provides an opportunity for you to ask questions about the classes or raise issues related to the points raised in this handout. You may find it useful, before you come for that interview, to make a note of the points that you wish to raise.

Good luck!

CHAPTER 6

❈

Automatic Pilot

SESSION I

From time to time, we all experience the effects of absent minded-
ness. We may read a whole page of a book and find that we have
taken in nothing. Or drive home along our normal route, only to arrive and realize that we had intended to stop and pick something up
at a friend's house that was out of the way. In such cases, we may or
may not have been aware of where our attention had gone.

When asked to describe these kinds of events, many people use
the term "automatic pilot" as a way of saying that they are just behaving mechanically, without really being aware of what is going on. In
automatic pilot mode, it is as if the body is doing one thing, while the
mind is doing something else. Most often, we do not intend to be
preoccupied with this or that—it simply happens. The mind is therefore passive much of the time, allowing itself to be "caught" by
thoughts, memories, plans, or feelings.

While, many times, we may not be fully aware of what is happening, this state of mind is especially problematic if we have suffered
from depression in the past. In automatic pilot, fragments of negative
thinking are less likely to be noticed. If unchecked, they may co-
alesce into patterns that lead to stronger feelings of sadness and more

BOX 6.1

⚯

Theme and Curriculum for Session 1

THEME

Mindfulness starts when we recognize the tendency to be on automatic pilot and make a commitment to learning how best to step out of it to become aware of each moment. Practice in purposely moving attention around the body shows both how simple and difficult this can be.

AGENDA

- Establish the orientation of the class.
- Set ground rules regarding confidentiality and privacy.
- Ask participants to pair up and introduce themselves to each other, then to the group as a whole.
- Raisin Exercise.
- Feedback and Discussion of Raisin Exercise.
- Body Scan Practice—starting with a short breath focus.
- Feedback and Discussion of Body Scan.
- Homework: Discuss and assign for the coming week:
  Body Scan Tape for 6 out of 7 days.
  Mindfulness of a routine activity.
- Distribute tapes and Session 1 participant handouts (including Homework Record Forms).
- End the class with a short breath focus, 2–3 minutes on the breath.

PLANNING AND PREPARATION

- In addition to your personal preparation before the class, remember to bring a bowl with raisins and a spoon, as well as copies of the Body Scan Tape.

PARTICIPANT HANDOUTS

Handout 6.1. A Definition of Mindfulness
Handout 6.2. Summary of Session 1: Automatic Pilot
Handout 6.3. Homework for Week Following Session 1
Handout 6.4. A Patient's Report
Handout 6.5. Homework Record Form—Session 1

severe depression. By the time the unwanted thoughts or feelings surface, they are often too strong to be dealt with easily. We have more to say about alternative ways of handling such thoughts and feelings later.

First however, we have to deal with the start of the sequence, the day-to-day "mindlessness" that seems harmless but can be so damaging if a person has a history of emotional problems. An important first step in helping recovered depressed patients stay well is to find ways of helping them recognize and then intentionally step out of automatic pilot mode. The practice of mindfulness involves becoming more aware of these patterns of the mind, so that we can learn to pay attention intentionally, that is, with awareness.

It is one thing to decide that a fundamental building block of preventing relapse is to teach people to recognize those times when their minds are running on automatic pilot and to teach them intentionally to shift their awareness to something else. It is quite another to find a simple way of showing this to people early on, in the first session, in a way that does not just add one more "wrong thing" they are doing.

When we first visited the Stress Reduction Clinic at UMass Medical Center, we sat in on Session 1 of a new class led by Jon Kabat-Zinn. After a short introductory talk reminding participants of why they had come, he asked people to introduce themselves, first in pairs and then to the whole class, saying their name, why they had come, and what they hoped to get out of the program. He then introduced a short meditation exercise that went to the heart of the automatic pilot theme. It involved eating a raisin, and after participating in the exercise ourselves, we did not hesitate to adopt it.

Eating is a particularly useful task to use for this first exercise because it is such an "automatic act," hardly ever done mindfully. It is therefore a good illustration of the extent to which we are often unaware of what is going on, as well as an example of the changes that can take place when we slow down such a simple act and focus on it. This simple eating exercise is a first step in helping participants understand what mindfulness is.

THE RAISIN EXERCISE

How much explanation should be given at the start of this exercise? It is most helpful to keep any explanations very brief: to err on the side of saying too little rather than too much. Our aim from the outset is to teach the course as experientially as possible; as with other practices in this program, participants learn from them by first having the experience and only afterwards trying to make sense of what it means. The transcript illustrates how we guide people through the raisin exercise.

The exercise is an excellent introduction to mindfulness for people who have been depressed. First, it provides an experiential rather than a verbal problem-solving base for learning. It sets a scene in which learning takes place through practice* and feedback from the practice. The practice is central and will become the core of the course. But the raisin exercise is also a very good introduction to the way in which we, as instructors, can most helpfully respond to what people say following the exercise. We need to embody in the way we deal with issues raised in the class the very approach to those issues we hope participants will find helpful. If we do not embody a spirit of genuine curiosity and inquiry about people's experience, or if we tend to rush for a premature explanation of what is going on, how can we expect participants to change the way they approach the tasks they are going to do? The hope is that, in time, a gradual tuning of people's experience might take place, and with it, the realization that one can practice mindfulness by being present in all waking moments, no matter how ordinary or routine.

One way to facilitate this is to ensure that as many questions as possible are open-ended (e.g., "What comments would anyone like to make about what we just did?"). This way of using the practice in the class is not easy to learn. Closed-ended questions come all too naturally ("Did anyone feel tired?", "Did your mind wander?"). Such closed questions produce, rather inevitably, a "yes" or "no" response.

---

*We use the word "practice" here to refer to the formal and informal mindfulness exercises that participants will be learning to use in their daily lives. Although it has this meaning, it retains its more usual meaning to convey the idea of a gentle and persistent attempt to learn a skill, or in this case, to become aware of a mode of mind.

BOX 6.2

⊗

Transcript: The Raisin Exercise

I'm going to go around the class and give you each a few objects.

Now, what I would like you to do is focus on one of the objects and just imagine that you have never seen anything like it before. Imagine you have just dropped in from Mars this moment and you have never seen anything like it before in your life.

Note. There is at least a 10-second pause between phrases, and the instructions are delivered in a matter-of-fact way, at a slow but deliberate pace, asking the class to do the following:

Taking one of these objects and holding it in the palm of your hand, or between your finger and thumb. (*Pause*)

Paying attention to seeing it. (*Pause*)

Looking at it carefully, as if you had never seen such a thing before. (*Pause*)

Turning it over between your fingers. (*Pause*)

Exploring its texture between your fingers. (*Pause*)

Examining the highlights where the light shines . . . the darker hollows and folds. (*Pause*)

Letting your eyes explore every part of it, as if you had never seen such a thing before. (*Pause*)

And if, while you are doing this, any thoughts come to mind about "what a strange thing we are doing" or "what is the point of this" or "I don't like these," then just noting them as thoughts and bringing your awareness back to the object. (*Pause*)

And now smelling the object, taking it and holding it beneath your nose, and with each inbreath, carefully noticing the smell of it. (*Pause*)

And now taking another look at it. (*Pause*)

And now slowly taking the object to your mouth, maybe noticing how your hand and arm know exactly where to put it, perhaps noticing your mouth watering as it comes up. (*Pause*)

And then gently placing the object in the mouth, noticing how it is "received," without biting it, just exploring the sensations of having it in your mouth. (*Pause*)

And when you are ready, very consciously taking a bite into it and noticing the tastes that it releases. (*Pause*)

(*cont.*)

Transcript: The Raisin Exercise (cont.)

Slowly chewing it, . . . noticing the saliva in the mouth, . . . the change in consistency of the object. (*Pause*)

Then, when you feel ready to swallow, seeing if you can first detect the intention to swallow as it comes up, so that even this is experienced consciously before you actually swallow it. (*Pause*)

Finally, seeing if you can follow the sensations of swallowing it, sensing it moving down to your stomach, and also realizing that your body is now exactly one raisin heavier.

Based on Kabat-Zinn.[64]

By contrast, look at the following response to a more open-ended question:

I: Does anyone want to say anything about their experiences while eating?

P: Different thoughts went through my mind, looking at the raisins.

I: Would you be able to say what kind of thoughts went through your mind?

P: I was thinking how strange that something quite so dried up and ordinary-looking could taste so good . . . that if we didn't know how it tasted, perhaps we wouldn't bother trying it.

I: So, thoughts associated with the raisin—where did those thoughts take you?

P: Different occasions—dried up deserts, hot sand . . . holidays with my parents when I was small—different associations.

I: That's interesting; that's really nice. So the task is to actually focus your awareness on the raisin, but the mind isn't having any of that!

P: It goes off in all sorts of directions.

I: It goes from the raisin to reflections on how curious that it should taste nice, and it's sort of dried up, to hot sand, to holidays with your parents. . . . It's a lovely example of the way the mind has its own agenda, if you like. The exercise is one where we're trying to focus our attention in the here and now, in this moment, and there we go—we're traveling back to sandy deserts, to your parents, to other places. The mind's gone off on its own. That's a very important thing to notice. We'll come back to that shortly. Any other comments?

Later, the instructor will be able to relate the participant's experience to the theme of the program: that the wandering mind during periods of automatic pilot can be particularly dangerous when mood is sinking, and associations and memories are likely to be depressing. It is therefore good to know what's going on in this stream of associations and to be able to disengage intentionally.

The raisin exercise also offers participants a direct sampling of a new way of relating to experience, contrasting it with the usual automatic pilot way of doing things. They find that paying attention in this way reveals unexpected little things about a raisin, such as its ridges, the folds in its skin, and the small scar at one end, where it was once connected to something larger than itself, that is, to the vine. Some say they can only think of how they like or how they dislike raisins. Others say that they are able to see the raisin with greater clarity, or that the raisin has a stronger, more vivid taste. We find that this aspect can be explored further by asking, "Did anyone notice anything different from the way you usually eat? What was the difference?" Participants most commonly point out the difference between the way they ate the raisin during the exercise and their normal way of eating.

P2: You wouldn't even stop to notice it. You'd just throw it in automatically. You wouldn't savor a raisin like that.

I: So you'd be quicker and more automatic? And what do you think would be the key differences between this experience and stuffing it in like that? What would you say you might notice?

P2: The *taste* more . . .

I: You noticed the taste more?

P2: And the texture. They were sort of dry on the outside and then you get into the more juicy bit, . . . I never noticed that before.

Another set of responses clearly show a growing awareness of the difference between this experience and what normally happens in everyday life.

I: How about the actual experience that you've all had? Any comments on that?

P3: I don't usually eat them; but for some reason, our cat loves raisins, so when I'm cooking, I throw a few down for her. I was thinking, actually, next time I give some to the cat, I think I'll have some. It was really nice doing it really slow. I liked that.

I: How was it different from the normal experience?

P3: Well, because I just normally shovel stuff in my mouth, you know, as quickly as possible, in order to go and do something else, really, like throwing coal onto a fire.

I: OK. So could you say a little bit more about how this was different?

P3: Well I *knew* I was eating it. That probably sounds a bit odd.

I: No, that's interesting. You knew you were . . .

P3: I knew I was eating it.

Note, here, that it is not clear whether the participant was using the word "know" to mean intellectual, factual knowledge or more direct sensory experience. Given the theme of the program—of moving away from rumination toward direct experience—this was an interesting thing to explore (though not necessarily to develop further at this point).

I: Could you say a little bit more about that?

P3: Well, I just think I was extremely aware of the fact that I was eating something.

I: Right. As a fact or as a sensation?

P3: As a sensation, yeah, definitely.

I: The taste or . . . ?

P3: Yeah, and all that stuff about your arm and everything. I just grab things usually. I don't know what my arms are doing normally; I mean, I know but I don't feel it.

I: That's a really really important distinction. So that, compared to the usual experience, there was much more awareness of direct experience.

P3: Yeah.

I: Direct experience of physical sensations in your arm, direct experience of the taste?

P3: Exactly.

I: OK, that's very helpful, thank you. Any other comments on the experience?

P4: I guess it was sensual, wasn't it? If I can remember what "sensual" is (*laughs*). Yeah, I think it could be described as being sensual.

I: Can you say a little bit more about what you mean?

P4: Well, I mean, I was thinking: I should do this more often because I'm actually experiencing something far more . . . um . . . in a sort of stronger way than usual awareness. I suppose, yeah, its sort of a sensual experience.

I: Right, rather than just some automatic experience that passes you by.

P4: Yes.

I: So these are really important points: that intentionally and deliberately bringing awareness to something changes the experience. It actually can enrich the experience, change the nature of the experience, and it makes you aware of things that often you may not have been aware of, like the sensations in your arm. Any other comments before we move on?

Of course, participants do not necessarily find the exercise enjoyable. The instructor still emphasizes the importance of noticing these reactions:

P5: I thought it was frustrating. Sitting here thinking . . .

I: That is very interesting. So the sort of thing that was running off in your mind was a sort of "Let's get on with it" kind of thing. "Why are we dragging this all out?" A real sense of frustration?

P5: Because I only eat when I am hungry.

I: OK, so that's interesting. Were you able to notice that and come back to the raisin?

P5: I could just come back and eat the raisin.

I: Good noticing. Anything else?

All these reactions, whether they appear to be positive or negative, are welcome. They can be woven into a more general "pulling together" of all the feedback comments in a way that draws out the relevance of becoming more aware to the aim of relapse prevention.

I: So really, this is a very simple exercise that is just meant to illustrate how, first of all, much of the time we are actually not getting our moments' worth, if you like. You know, all that taste, all that smell, all the visual patterns of the texture, you know, they just disappear in one handful. We are not really there for it. And it also shows what happens when we bring awareness to experiences in a different way. This, for most of us, is slightly different from the way we normally eat raisins. It is interesting that it provides a sort of background against which we can then begin to notice any sense of irritation, urgency, wanting to get on, "what on earth are we doing this for?" So it's all good noticing.

This exercise is an example of a lot of what we will be doing. We will practice bringing awareness to our everyday activities, so that we know what is going on and can actually change the nature of the experience. If you are fully aware of thoughts, feelings, sensations in the body, in the sense that you may have glimpsed in this raisin exercise, you can actually change the experience; you have got more choices, more freedom. At the moment, this is just theoretical; we need to have more and more experiences of bringing awareness to bear, so that you can see, eventually, in what way it is going to help. And that's why I am asking you, for the moment, to take an interest in what happens when you do something simple like this. At the moment, the connection between slowly eating a raisin and protecting yourself against depression in the future may not be obvious. But the first step, and what we are doing in the first part of the program, is really training awareness.

So the basic take-home message from that little exercise is that we're not aware of what's going on a lot of the time. If we can bring awareness we become aware of aspects of life that otherwise may just slide by us, both the good and the bad. Missing out on the good means that life isn't as rich as it might be. Not being aware of the bad means that we're not in a position to actually take skillful action ourselves. Depression can creep up on us when our minds are elsewhere.

We can't actually control what comes into the mind, but what we can control is what we do next, the next step. And this program is all about being able to move to a place of awareness from which we can choose what the next step is, rather than run off the old habits of mind.

In fact, participants in the classes find it relatively easy to use their experiences with the raisin exercise to draw out its relevance to their tendency to fall back into depressive mind states. First, when they start paying attention a little more closely to experience in this way, they discover quite powerfully, for themselves how much they normally do automatically; how much of the time the mind is more likely to be in the past or future than in the present; how, in any moment, most of us are only partially aware of what is actually occurring. Whereas many people might sometimes have noticed the effects of being on automatic pilot (e.g., most of them related easily to the example of driving their car for miles without realizing where their mind had been), it still comes as a discovery for them to see how the same tendency is present for much of everyday life.

Second, the exercise shows how paying attention in a particular way (that is, intentionally, in the present moment and without judgment) can actually change the nature of the experience. By simply paying attention, people find it possible both to wake themselves up from automatic pilot mode and to connect more fully with the present. As participants find when they eat one raisin mindfully, there is often more that awaits us in the present than we imagine, especially if we have been operating automatically a good deal of the time. Through exercises such as that with the raisin, participants are able to come to this realization, not because the instructor tells them, but through their own discovery.

TRAINING IN AWARENESS: USING THE BODY AS A FOCUS

Much emphasis in MBCT is placed on providing participants with opportunities to relate mindfully and directly to their experience. The next stage of Session 1 builds on the raisin exercise, as participants start to explore the awareness of bodily sensations using a practice called the "body scan." A major aim of the body scan practice is to bring detailed awareness to each part of the body. It is where participants first learn to keep their attention focused over a sustained period of time, and it also serves to help them develop concentration, calmness, flexibility of attention, and mindfulness. It gives an opportunity to practice bringing a particular quality of awareness to things (in this case, the body), an awareness characterized by gentleness and curiosity.

Why use the body as the first object of attention? First, because a greater awareness of the body will be helpful in learning how better to deal with emotion. Powerful feelings such as sadness or hopelessness can be expressed not only as thoughts or mental events but also as effects in the body. Stooped posture, heaviness in the chest, or tightness in the shoulders may at times signal the presence of strong feelings of which we are not fully aware. What happens in the body importantly affects what happens in the mind. Feedback on how the body feels is often an integral part of the loops that sustain old habits of thinking and feeling.

Second, people who have been depressed very often try to *think* their way out of troubling feelings. An alternative is to bring awareness to manifestations of emotion as physical sensations or felt senses *in* the body. In time, this allows a shift of the center of gravity of attention away from "being in the head," toward an awareness of the body. It offers the prospect of coming at emotion from a fresh perspective, honing in on a new aspect: "How am I feeling this in my body?"

We introduce the body scan as an exercise in awareness, in which we invite people to move their attention intentionally around the body, and to discover what happens when they do so. A helpful way of introducing the body scan is to follow the MBSR approach of linking it to the raisin exercise that participants have just completed. Just as paying attention has allowed participants to relate directly and in a new way to their experience of eating a raisin, the same can be done with physical sensations. The key issue in doing the body scan is awareness of physical sensations in the body, bringing the same quality of direct awareness as in the raisin exercise.

To begin the body scan, we simply ask participants to lie on their backs, usually on a mat or soft surface (see Box 6.3 for step-by-step instructions). Next, we spend a few minutes focusing on the movement of the breath into and out of the body. Then, we give the instructions for the body scan: Participants are asked to move their minds through the different regions of the body. The aim is to bring awareness intentionally to each region of the body in turn, exploring the actual physical sensations that are present in that region at that moment. During the 40 to 45 minutes it takes to complete the body scan, participants have many opportunities to practice its basic instructions—to bring awareness to a particular region of the body, to hold it in awareness for a short time, and finally to release and "let go" of that region before moving their attention to the next region.

CREATING A CONTEXT FOR FORMAL MINDFULNESS PRACTICE: GENERAL COMMENTS

Several general issues arise when starting formal mindfulness practice. Since these start to occur with the introduction of the body scan, we mention them here. First, there is the issue of success and failure. It is important to mention that there is no success or failure involved.

BOX 6.3

⚛

Body Scan Meditation

1. Lie down, making yourself comfortable, lying on your back on a mat or rug on the floor or on your bed, in a place where you will be warm and undisturbed. Allow your eyes to close gently.

2. Take a few moments to get in touch with the movement of your breath and the sensations in the body. When you are ready, bring your awareness to the physical sensations in your body, especially to the sensations of touch or pressure, where your body makes contact with the floor or bed. On each outbreath, allow yourself to let go, to sink a little deeper into the mat or bed.

3. Remind yourself of the intention of this practice. Its aim is not to feel any different, relaxed, or calm; this may happen or it may not. Instead, the intention of the practice is, as best you can, to bring awareness to any sensations you detect, as you focus your attention on each part of the body in turn.

4. Now bring your awareness to the physical sensations in the lower abdomen, becoming aware of the changing patterns of sensations in the abdominal wall as you breathe in, and as you breathe out. Take a few minutes to feel the sensations as you breathe in and as you breathe out.

5. Having connected with the sensations in the abdomen, bring the focus or "spotlight" of your awareness down the left leg, into the left foot, and out to the toes of the left foot. Focus on each of the toes of the left foot in turn, bringing a gentle curiosity to investigate the quality of the sensations you find, perhaps noticing the sense of contact between the toes, a sense of tingling, warmth, or no particular sensation.

6. When you are ready, on an inbreath, feel or imagine the breath entering the lungs, and then passing down into the abdomen, into the left leg, the left foot, and out to the toes of the left foot. Then, on the outbreath, feel or imagine the breath coming all the way back up, out of the foot, into the leg, up through the abdomen, chest, and out through the nose. As best you can, continue this for a few breaths, breathing down into the toes, and back out from the toes. It may be difficult to get the hang of this—just practice this "breathing into" as best you can, approaching it playfully.

(cont.)

7. Now, when you are ready, on an outbreath, let go of awareness of the toes, and bring your awareness to the sensations on the bottom of your left foot—bringing a gentle, investigative awareness to the sole of the foot, the instep, the heel (e.g., noticing the sensations where the heel makes contact with the mat or bed). Experiment with "breathing with" the sensations—being aware of the breath in the background, as, in the foreground, you explore the sensations of the lower foot.

8. Now allow the awareness to expand into the rest of the foot—to the ankle, the top of the foot, and right into the bones and joints. Then, taking a slightly deeper breath, directing it down into the whole of the left foot, and, as the breath lets go on the outbreath, let go of the left foot completely, allowing the focus of awareness to move into the lower left leg—the calf, shin, knee, and so on, in turn.

9. Continue to bring awareness, and a gentle curiosity, to the physical sensations in each part of the rest of the body in turn—to the upper left leg, the right toes, right foot, right leg, pelvic area, back, abdomen, chest, fingers, hands, arms, shoulders, neck, head, and face. In each area, as best you can, bring the same detailed level of awareness and gentle curiosity to the bodily sensations present. As you leave each major area, "breathe in" to it on the inbreath, and let go of that region on the outbreath.

10. When you become aware of tension, or of other intense sensations in a particular part of the body, you can "breathe in" to them—using the inbreath gently to bring awareness right into the sensations, and, as best you can, have a sense of their letting go, or releasing, on the outbreath.

11. The mind will inevitably wander away from the breath and the body from time to time. That is entirely normal. It is what minds do. When you notice it, gently acknowledge it, noticing where the mind has gone off to, and then gently return your attention to the part of the body you intended to focus on.

12. After you have "scanned" the whole body in this way, spend a few minutes being aware of a sense of the body as a whole, and of the breath flowing freely in and out of the body.

13. If you find yourself falling asleep, you might find it helpful to prop your head up with a pillow, open your eyes, or do the practice sitting up rather than lying down.

The problem is how to do this in a way that does not put the thought of success into people's heads. An understandable reaction to such practice, particularly for people who have suffered from depression, is to seek social approval and/or seek to achieve "high marks." Many depressive habits of mind revolve around the themes of performance/ achievement or social evaluation, so people who have been depressed naturally bring this attitude to bear on any task. The body scan task is not immune to these attitudes, nor is any other practice during or after the 8 weeks of classes. Of course, we also recognized this tendency in ourselves. Success–failure ("Am I doing this right?") and approval issues ("Will people think I'm all right?") are likely to surface again and again. The task is not to try and stop such thoughts from arising, but to learn to recognize them when they come, so that we might respond to them skillfully.

We therefore find it helpful to mention over and over again that "doing it well" is not the issue. We follow other mindfulness teachers in including, early on in the instructions, "It is important not to try too hard" and "We are not trying to achieve any special state; we are not even trying to relax." Later in the instructions, the theme is again picked up: "sometimes the practice may bring up discomfort or boredom. If this happens, it does not mean that you have failed." We offer encouragement by being curious about what such discomfort or boredom feels like in the body, what sensation accompanies each emotion.

A second, major general issue is how to respond when difficulties occur. For example, in the body scan, some participants find that they or their neighbor cannot stay awake. Others find that sensations of physical discomfort distract them from the task. Despite this, the spirit embodied by the instructor remains "Whatever happens, whatever comes up, that is OK." Over time, one is able to see such difficulties as opportunities to bring awareness to these feelings and sensations rather than worrying about them, or letting them take control. The essence of the approach is to understand that these reactions are going to come up anyway, since they are part and parcel of life itself. It is how one handles them that makes the difference—whether or not they rule our lives to an inordinate degree.

The instructor has the opportunity to embody this sense of curiosity and adventure in the way he or she handles issues that arise in the class. Right from the start of doing MBCT with participants, we became aware of a wish to make things better for participants, to help them fix their problem, and to reduce the pain of their emotional upset. When we were not thinking how good it would be to make people better, we found ourselves wanting to explain the theory to them. As scientists, we get very excited about theory! In time, we found that there was no need to rush things, that each of these elements had their place. Sometimes it felt appropriate to take a very pragmatic approach in dealing with difficulties that arose, and, at other times, to explain about depression and its nature. But our primary emphasis was on evoking a sense of curiosity in participants, and on developing their intentional awareness of sensations in each moment.

Along with any physical sensations that participants notice in particular body regions, they may also become aware of negative, judgmental thoughts or emotions. Despite our instructions during the practice, some participants found it very difficult to let go of the tendency to check how well they were doing. Thoughts about how they looked, what parts of their bodies they wanted to change, or feelings of embarrassment and awkwardness often came to mind when they focused on the body in this way. We emphasized that one approach is to acknowledge the feelings and bring to them a sense of curiosity and a willingness to observe. This provides an initial opportunity to relate to thoughts and feelings as mind states rather than to "be" or identify with them. Such experiences can be used to teach one of the core messages of MBCT, namely, that it is both possible and something of an adventure in self-discovery to learn that, through becoming aware we can relate quite differently to our thoughts, feelings, perceptions, and impulses—in other words, to our experience of being alive.

REACTIONS AND RESPONSES

In the examples that follow, notice how commonly participants interpreted the instructions as rules to follow (rules that they found themselves or others breaking): rules such as "Don't move or fidget,"

"Don't go to sleep" (Participant 1); "Don't open your eyes or let your mind wander" (Participant 2); "Relax!" (Participant 3); "Don't get out of time with the tape" (Participant 4). Note how each, in his or her own way, moved rapidly from an observation about what was happening, to a negative and self-critical judgment.

P: My legs felt really heavy to start with, and then I couldn't keep them still. I wanted to keep moving them all the time. I thought there must be something wrong because I couldn't hear anybody else moving and I was desperate to move mine. And then I heard somebody beginning to snore gently, and I thought: *Oh, my gosh. This is awful. Somebody has gone to sleep.*

I: Wonderful, wonderful.

P: I was really worried about it, because they had gone to sleep. I thought: *Please don't go to sleep.*

I: This is great. I am really glad you are saying all this. This is wonderful. Because the whole point of this is that we become aware of whatever is. So that there isn't a right or a wrong thing to happen. The aim of the exercise is, as best you can (and it is difficult), becoming aware of whatever you are feeling at the time. And for you—your fidgetiness and wanting to move—that's great. It's just your experience in that moment. It's not wrong. It's not what shouldn't happen. That is the thing to become aware of. And eventually, you know, with that awareness, you may be able to become aware of the urge to move and make a decision, whether you are going to go with it or not.

P: I tried to suppress it. I wanted to sort of move around.

I: OK, well, there is no need to try and fight these things. This is hard, particularly for something as strong as an agitation. But, as best you can, just acknowledge it: "Right, OK, there you are. I really want to get up and jump around here, and I am fed up with this. It's going too slowly." Whatever. As best you can, acknowledge all of it. Because that is your experience in that moment, and that is what you really need to know. So you acknowledge it, you don't push it away. Acknowledge it, and then, as best you can, bring your attention back to whatever bit of the body we are on.

P2: My arms felt ever so itchy. I kept getting midges [flies] going round me. There was one on the table and twice it went on my arm, and I opened my eye and had a look. I didn't think I was supposed to do that.

P3: I kept thinking I am supposed to be relaxed here.

I: OK. So this thing that we are going to come across over and over again is this idea of "how things are meant to be" or "how things should be." And it's this tension that causes our distress. It is often something that was put in our minds as children. It may have been useful then, but it may not be useful now. And if we can become aware of this, then we can let go of it and just deal with what is. How do we do this? By becoming aware of the feeling that "I should be doing this right," acknowledging it, and letting go of it. Then we are dealing with reality, with actuality in this moment, rather than all these images about what should be or ought to be, or what we ought to expect.

P4: I find it hard to breathe out when told to. I keep getting it back to front. My breath was not in time with the instructions.

I: Just see if you can be gentle with yourself. See if you can cultivate this attitude, not "It's wrong and naughty; I'm doing it back to front" but "Oh, that's how it is."

In each case, notice how the response of the instructor invites people to acknowledge and become curious about the things that come up for them, to be gentle with themselves rather than blaming themselves for having failed. The task is like that of a cartographer making a map of relatively unexplored land. Whatever the cartographer finds, whether the view is of rolling hills or dangerous-looking precipices, the task is the same: to note as accurately as possible what is there. *As best you can, acknowledge all of it. Because that is your experience in that moment, and that is what you really need to know.*

LEARNING THROUGH HOMEWORK

Homework is a routine aspect of MBCT. The kind of knowledge that we can get from talking about things is of only limited use for our purposes. The real business in MBCT is learning by doing, and in order to learn, we need to do. This is why the homework is so central and not an optional extra. We give participants daily, formal meditation practice as homework that consists of audiotaped guided meditation instructions. These tapes are also used in the UMass MBSR program. The tapes come in two series, both recorded by Jon Kabat-Zinn. Series 1 consists of two 45-minute taped instructions for a guided body scan and a guided meditation on the breath, body, sounds, thoughts, and choiceless awareness. There are also two different sessions of guided hatha yoga. Tape 1 of Series 1 is distributed for homework in this first session. The formal homework also includes keeping a written diary of the daily mindfulness practice on the Homework Record Form—Session 1 (Handout 6.5; also see other participant handouts for details of the homework for each session).

From the outset, we attempt to convey how serious we are about homework by making sure that enough time is left toward the end of the class to discuss the assignments for the coming week. We find that allowing sufficient time is important because there are often tapes and handouts to be distributed. All the homework assignments are listed on handouts, together with a summary of each session. We distribute the relevant handouts during each session, rather than giving everything at Session 1. Our reasoning is that "looking ahead" to what is to be done in future classes is not helpful to participants and might undermine the theme of awareness in the present moment.

All participants attend individual preclass interviews with the instructor, who emphasizes that "because the patterns of mind that we will be working to change have been around a long time, the mindfulness approach depends entirely on your willingness to do homework between class meetings." Each person is reminded that the commitment to spend time on homework is an essential part of the class. If participants do not feel able to make that commitment, it is better not to start the classes at that time.

Almost without exception, participants accept the need to do homework in principle but come up against a stumbling block once they start to consider how actually to do it. Some participants have very practical questions, for example, about the best time of day, the best place, and the particular type of equipment to use. Others express a sense that finding time is going to be very difficult, or that homework will take important time away from their families. We find that a useful, general approach is to encourage people to discover what works best for them, without compromising the commitment each of them has made at the start of the program to do the prescribed practice 6 days a week. We make a point of helping participants create a space for their practice by asking them whether they have a quiet place where they can do the practice. Is there a time when they will not be interrupted? What things do they think might get in the way of doing the homework? How do they intend to continue the homework through weekends, holidays, or when they have visitors?

"About the homework, there may be difficulties. Let me say two things. First, you will see in the handouts a report of someone who said, 'I couldn't do this. It went up and down, but eventually something seemed to happen,' so just hang on in there. Second, we asked members of the class who had come back for a follow-up meeting, having been through it themselves for 8 weeks, and with some time to look back on it, what single piece of advice they would offer to this new group starting today. With one voice they said, 'whatever happens, stick with it.' That may not seem relevant to you now, but it may be at some point. Remember, you do not have to enjoy it, you just have to do it."

MINDFULNESS OF EVERYDAY ACTIVITIES

We give participants daily formal practice as homework, and we also give some informal assignments. The idea is to enable participants to generalize to everyday life what they learn in the formal practice. For example, we asked people to perform an everyday activity mindfully. This simply involved choosing one routine activity and making a deliberate effort to bring moment-to-moment awareness to the activity, much as was done in the raisin exercise. Any activity—brushing one's teeth, taking a shower, or even taking out the garbage—will do. We stressed the importance of actually bringing oneself back into the moment, of being fully present, feeling the brush on the teeth or the water as it splashes on the back.

This type of moment-by-moment awareness helps us to mark the difference between being on automatic pilot and knowing what we are doing while we are actually doing it. Using it with routine activities also illustrates that there is nothing special about mindfulness. We can access it in the middle of whatever we are doing, just by choosing to pay attention.

ENDING THE CLASS

By the end of the first class, participants have been exposed to a lot of new information over a fairly short period of time. In starting work of this kind, they experience many different reactions to the ideas that have been introduced. Some of these reactions have been expressed; many have not. These and other experiences continue to surface over the coming weeks and become the material around which teaching takes place.

We find that the end of the session is a good time to provide the class with a summary of the session in a way that ties the strands together. We use the Summary of Session 1 (Handout 6.2) as the structure for this summary, directing participants' attention to the handouts as we summarize.

Finally, we end the class with a short 2- to 3-minute breath focus. Participants are invited to sit with their backs straight (but not stiff), and after a few moments, to focus their attention on their breath as it enters and leaves the body, noticing any sensations associated with it. It is a way to "ground" the class following the discussion, and to provide a foretaste of things to come.

⁜

A Definition of Mindfulness

Mindfulness means paying attention in a particular way:
on purpose,
in the present moment,
and nonjudgmentally.

—JON KABAT-ZINN

✇

Summary of Session 1: Automatic Pilot

In a car, we can sometimes drive for miles "on automatic pilot," without really being aware of what we are doing. In the same way, we may not be really "present," moment-by-moment, for much of our lives: We can often be "miles away" without knowing it.

On automatic pilot, we are more likely to have our "buttons pressed": Events around us and thoughts, feelings, and sensations in the mind (of which we may be only dimly aware) can trigger old habits of thinking that are often unhelpful and may lead to worsening mood.

By becoming more aware of our thoughts, feelings, and body sensations, from moment to moment, we give ourselves the possibility of greater freedom and choice; we do not have to go into the same old "mental ruts" that may have caused problems in the past.

The aim of this program is to increase awareness so that we can respond to situations with choice rather than react automatically. We do that by practicing to become more aware of where our attention is, and deliberately changing the focus of attention, over and over again.

To begin with, we use attention to different parts of the body as a focus to anchor our awareness in the moment. We will also be training ourselves to put attention and awareness in different places at will. This is the aim of the body scan exercise that is the main homework for next week.

⚽

Homework for Week Following Session 1

1. Do the Body Scan Tape (Tape 1, Side 1) six times before we meet again. Don't expect to feel anything in particular from listening to the tape. In fact, give up all expectations about it. Just let your experience be your experience. Don't judge it. Just keep doing it, and we'll talk about it next week.

2. Record on the Homework Record Form each time you listen to the tape. Also, make a note of anything that comes up in the homework, so that we can talk about it at the next meeting.

3. Choose one routine activity in your daily life and make a deliberate effort to bring moment-to-moment awareness to that activity each time you do it, just as we did in the raisin exercise. Possibilities include waking up in the morning, brushing your teeth, showering, drying your body, getting dressed, eating, driving, taking out the rubbish (garbage), shopping, and so on. Simply zero in on *knowing what you are doing as you are actually doing it.*

4. Note any times when you find yourself able to notice what you eat, in the same way you noticed the raisin.

5. Eat at least one meal "mindfully," in the way that you ate the raisin.

This patient had been hospitalized for depression 4 years before, following which her husband and children left her. There had been no further contact except through lawyers. She had become very depressed and lonely, although she had not been in the hospital again. Now over the worst of her depression, she started to use the Body Scan Tape to help prevent her mood from deteriorating. These were her comments looking back after 8 weeks:

"For the first 10 days it was like a burden. I kept 'wandering off' and then I would worry about whether I was doing it right. For example, I kept having flights of fantasy. When the tape mentioned Massachusetts, I would think of a trip to Boston with the family 5 years ago. My mind was all over the place. I tried too hard to stop it, I think.

"Another problem at the start was him saying, 'Just accept things as they are now.' I thought that was totally unreasonable. I thought to myself, 'I can't do that.'

"Eventually, I just put the tape on and expected to go off into a realm of thoughts. I didn't worry if concerns came in. Gradually, the 40 minutes passed without me losing him, and from then on, the next time was more effective.

"After 10 days, I relaxed more. I stopped worrying if I was thinking about anything else. When I stopped worrying about it, then I actually stopped the flights of fancy. If I did think of something else, I picked up the tape again when I stopped thinking. Gradually, the flights of fantasy reduced. I was happy to listen to him, and then I started to get some value from it.

"Soon I had developed it so that I could actually feel the breath going down to the base of my foot. Sometimes I didn't feel anything, but then I thought, 'If there's no feeling, then I can be satisfied with the fact there is no feeling.'

"It's not something you can do half a dozen times. It's got to be a daily thing. It becomes more real the more that you try it. I began to look forward to it.

"If people have got to structure the time for the 45 minutes for their tape, it may be easier to structure other things in their life as well. The tape, in itself, would prove an impetus."

☒

Homework Record Form—Session 1

Name: _____

Record on the Homework Record Form each time you practice. Also, make a note of anything that comes up in the homework, so that we can talk about it at the next meeting.

Day/date	Practice (Yes/No)	Comments
Wednesday Date:		
Thursday Date:		
Friday Date:		
Saturday Date:		
Sunday Date:		
Monday Date:		
Tuesday Date:		
Wednesday Date:		

CHAPTER 7

⚒

Dealing with Barriers

SESSION 2

All the people who come to the classes have made an enormous commitment. The diversity of reactions to the first full week of practice is equally enormous. For some, the challenge will have seemed too strong. They have had "an awful week," an awfulness compounded by their disappointment that this approach appears not to be helping or even to be making things worse. For others, it may have "gone very well"; they may have found the Body Scan Tape very relaxing. How can an instructor remain open and evenhanded in the light of all these different reactions?

When, in 1992, we started wondering whether mindfulness might be combined with cognitive therapy, we were helped to get a flavor of the Stress Reduction Clinic at the UMass Medical Center through a recent Public Broadcasting Service documentary that had been made about it. It followed a new class of participants as they attended the eight sessions and learned the mindfulness approach. In Session 1, we saw a sample of the instructor's initial remarks, his introduction of the raisin exercise, and the body scan. The program followed some of the participants home as they did the body scan practice for themselves on a daily basis. For the following week's session, the television program went directly from participants doing their homework practice to pictures of them arriving for Session 2, and giving their feedback on how the week's practice had gone. We were very interested in seeing how the instructor handled the very different reactions to the first week's tape. Only later, after we had visited and sampled the program for ourselves, did we realize that the inevitable pressure to condense 8 weeks into a 40-minute television program had meant that an important component had been left on the cutting room floor—the initial practice at the start of the session.

But not just the constraints of television forced the pace in this way. When participants arrived for the second session, both they and the instructor may have felt a strong need to share their experiences of the week. Before the session started, the room was filled with people talking and comparing notes. Participants knew a bit more about each other and, of course, they had just spent a week engaged in a new and unfamiliar practice. It was tempting then to follow the television editor and cut directly to discussion of how the week had gone for each of them. Indeed, this would have been an important part of a cognitive therapy approach—set the agenda for the session, then check how the homework has gone and what has been learned from it. This is a natural way to proceed if the task is to solve problems. Lay out the problems, then work as collaboratively as possible to find solutions.

We discovered that the mindfulness approach is radically different from the approach we might have used before. It does not provide a solution to anyone's problems, including depression. We found from the outset that, with MBCT, it is better not to start a class with discussion, but with practice. So, first thing, in each session, from Session 2 onward, the instructor leads the class in practice. Formal practice becomes the foundation on which the remainder of the class is built. In the case of Session 2, this is the body scan. Given the importance of allowing participants to become more aware of a different mode, the mode of "being" rather than "doing," starting with practice aims to help participants focus on the present moment.

None of these comments should be taken to imply that there is no agenda for each session. There is work to be done, and some effort is required to stay focused enough to use every moment of the 2 hours to give participants opportunities to experience how mindfulness might be relevant to their lives.

BOX 7.1

⊗

Theme and Curriculum for Session 2

THEME

Further focus on the body begins to show more clearly the chatter of the mind, and how it tends to control our reactions to everyday events.

AGENDA

- Body Scan Practice.
- Practice Review.
- Homework Review.
- Thoughts and Feelings Exercise ("Walking down the street"),
- Pleasant Events Calendar.
- Ten- to 15-minute sitting meditation.
- Distribute Session 2 participant handouts.
- Homework assignment:
  Body Scan Tape, 6 out of 7 days.
  Ten to 15 minutes of mindfulness of the breath, 6 out of 7 days.
  Pleasant Events Calendar (daily).
  Mindfulness of a routine activity.

PLANNING AND PREPARATION

- In addition to your personal preparation, bring a black or white board and markers for the Thoughts and Feelings Exercise.

PARTICIPANT HANDOUTS FOR SESSION 2

Handout 7.1. Summary of Session 2: Dealing with Barriers.
Handout 7.2. Tips for the Body Scan.
Handout 7.3. Mindfulness of the Breath.
Handout 7.4. The Breath.
Handout 7.5. Homework for Week Following Session 2.
Handout 7.6. Homework Record Form—Session 2.
Handout 7.7. Pleasant Events Calendar.

PRACTICE AS THE FOUNDATION
FOR THE CLASS

Session 2 aims to do a number of things to help people deal with any barriers they have encountered. First, we do the body scan practice, so that participants can once again shift from the mode of doing to simply being. Second, we use this practice as the basis for reviewing how things are going for participants, starting with the experience of the practice just completed, then moving to the experience of the formal and informal practice they have done during the week. This is important, since things that come up during the practice (e.g., a tendency to judge how it is going) touch on themes that will likely surface again in subsequent practice.

A third aim for the session is to show how depression creates difficulties in the way even mildly depressive thoughts and feelings feed off each other to create vicious spirals. The ease with which depressive interpretations can set off such spirals makes them seem hard to deal with in the practice. Helping people deal with them involves bringing participants to a point where they may see this process occurring more clearly for themselves. We seek to focus on this early in the classes, partly because of its centrality to the prevention of relapse (see Chapter 2), and partly because it might raise participants' level of motivation for persisting with the practice. This is because the old and very familiar mental habits of rumination will very commonly arise when doing the practice, and the pull they have on our attention illustrates well their power.

So we start with the body scan, followed by discussion of the practice. Responses to the practice are always varied. Some people fold new experiences of the practice just completed into their comments, while others want to discuss their experience of having done the body scan homework over the past week. We find it helpful to start discussion by staying as close as possible to feedback on the practice that has just ended. This involves postponing discussion of the homework until later in the session. The themes that commonly emerge from the practice in the session match very well participants' experience during the week. The most common themes that come out of the practice in the session are "Am I doing it right?," "I get discomfort when I do it," "The conditions aren't right," and "My mind just keeps wandering." We describe these first, before discussing the themes that emerge more specifically from the homework.

Let us start with the experience of one participant, Louise, giving a little of her background to set the context.

Louise was 38 years old when she was referred to the MBCT program. She had been depressed on and off for many years, with the last episode stretching over 9 months. She came because she feared that her episodes of depression were getting more severe. She was feeling better at the time she was referred to the MBCT trial (recall that MBCT was devised specifically for people who are not depressed at the moment but remain vulnerable to future depression). Louise had a husband and three children, and worked as a school receptionist. When Louise was a child, her perfectionist parents sent her to a convent school (the family was Roman Catholic). Louise often felt she was a poor mother and wife. When she was depressed, her lack of energy confirmed to her how bad she was, and she ruminated endlessly about this.

At the preclass interview, the instructor was able to link some of the core themes of the program to Louise's particular experience. For example, she knew that she judged herself too harshly. She knew this "intellectually" but had not been able to do anything about it. Similarly, she recognized how easily her moods were triggered. Once again, knowledge of this had not altered the pattern. She talked of an "avalanche" effect . . . a "slippery slope," and the instructor talked about how difficult it can be to see the "warning signs."

At this interview, the instructor also took time to explain MBCT—the 8-week, 2 hours a week commitment. Homework was particularly emphasized. If Louise was not sure she could find the time for this right now, it might be better not to start the classes, because the homework was such an important component. This did not put her off. (It rarely puts anyone off. Most people can see that some work will be necessary, but, once the work starts, they may have very different reactions.)

ATTITUDE TOWARD THE PRACTICE:
"AM I DOING IT RIGHT?"

Louise found that she could concentrate on the body scan in the session much better than she had during the week. As the session progressed, we were able to build up a picture of the nature of this difference. During the week, Louise had listened to the tapes "religiously." She said she tried to relax but any distraction made her angry and upset, and this was not the "way it should be." Even worse, Louise found that as she moved attention around her body, she noticed a lot of tension: tightness in the chest, stiffness in the lower back, tension in the shoulders. Her discomfort was compounded by another feeling: If it did not feel pleasant, then she must not be doing it right. This theme ("Am I doing it right?") connects with what a lot of people in the class feel at some point. For some, it is pain. For others, it is that they fall asleep, lose concentration, keep thinking of other things or focusing on the wrong part of the body, or have no sensations whatsoever. There are a million ways in which people can think they are getting it wrong. The mindfulness approach allows people to experience these feelings in the moment, to acknowledge and register them as events in the mind, and continue with the exercise. Recall the instruction given at the end of the first session: You do not have to enjoy it, just do it! In Louise's case, there was also a specific problem of pain and discomfort, and it is to this that we now turn.

PAINFUL SENSATIONS

Louise's reaction to her pain is a common one and provides an important opportunity for new learning. The intention in the body scan includes paying attention to physical sensations in the body. When strong sensations are present, then the task remains the same, simply, to bring awareness to that region and, as best we can, note carefully the sensations that arise. This involves assuming a different stance than the one we habitually take. A typical reaction is to start thinking *about* the pain. This is what had happened to Louise. In answer to a question about what had gone through her mind when she had noticed these strong sensations, she said: "It was really uncomfortable. Why am I so tense? Why can't I do anything right?" In the ensuing inner monologue, Louise had, in effect, added concepts to the experience in an understandable attempt to find a way to reduce the discomfort. The problem was that in doing so she had wandered away from the current focus and made the experience something other than what it was. What began as an uncomfortable sensation was now an inner monologue about stress at work, tensions with her husband and children, and Louise wondered why she couldn't cope better with it all.

After a number of questions about how long the feelings of discomfort had lasted and whether they had stayed the same or changed over time, the instructor invited Louise, when next she noticed her mind beginning to wander in this way, to bring awareness back as best she could to the part of the body currently under focus in the body scan, that is, to begin to practice untangling herself from the knots that the monologue was busy creating.

Recall that Louise reported that practice was easier in the class than at home. This a common reaction. It is, in one sense, good that people see the classes as a "safe haven," but it also raises an interesting issue—how to meditate when conditions are not so conducive.

"THE CONDITIONS WEREN'T RIGHT"

One of the most compelling obstructions to using the approaches we speak about in this book is the idea that conditions have to be right. The idea is that we may be able to use this approach to deal with things when we are reasonably calm, or have the time, or when there are no distractions, but otherwise, it just does not work so well.

At one of the first MBCT classes held at Cambridge during the development of MBCT, the cleaning staff were working outside the meeting room. The noise of one person calling to another was followed by a vacuum cleaner being switched on, and then the drone of the machine as it did its work out in the hallway.

In the review of the practice later on, much of the discussion focused on the noise. Some participants found they were able to weave the cleaners' noise into the fabric of the awareness of sounds in general. For others, however, the noise was experienced as a distraction from the task of sitting quietly. They found it difficult not to get annoyed, thinking that they were being needlessly disturbed.

As the class continued to explore these different perspectives, one thing emerged that seemed important: All who heard the cleaners were also aware of some negative thoughts or reactions. After all, "Didn't they see the sign on the door that indicated a class was in progress?" Some people were able to note these thoughts, let them go, and return to the practice. It was as if they came to see the cleaners' noise as part of the exercise and were able to let go of the need for conditions to be other than they were. What seemed to fuel other class members' reactions was the expectation that this sitting should be a certain way, and that it was turning out to be different than they had hoped. This second, more angry reaction, is quite normal; it does not require immediate remedial action, as if these participants are somehow inadequate in their practice. This frustration happens, and it happens to people who have been practicing for years. The cleaners' noises created a great opportunity to notice what happens when things do not go as planned.

No therapy or meditation will prevent unpleasant things from happening in our daily lives, and these, together with the mood changes that accompany them, will feature as much (perhaps more) when doing the practice as at other times. For people who have been depressed in the past, such occasions are times when the mood could begin to "lock into" the self-perpetuating pattern mentioned earlier. The rumination starts, and the repetitive thoughts may be far more troubling than the vacuum cleaner that the participants experienced in the class. Distraction caused by external factors and mind wandering are constant themes. Such mind wandering often has a theme of disappointed expectations, including disappointment about the practice itself not proceeding as it should. Many participants believe that it would be easier to deal with any discomfort and other difficulties with the practice if the mind were not so often distracted from the point of focus in the exercise. This raises a more general question that many people bring up again and again: what to do when the mind wanders.

MIND WANDERING AND REPETITIVE HABITS OF MIND

Both in our own experience and in that of others, we find that mind wandering is often regarded as a "mistake" that needs correction. But "wandering" is what minds do. It is their nature to wander, and we cannot stop them from doing so. The issue is how we relate to their wanderings. When we see our task as trying to empty the mind or stop our thoughts, or to make the mind blank, and a thought occurs, we tend to see it as something that has gone wrong and needs remedial correction. Even very skilled meditation teachers, who have been practicing for years, find they have thoughts going through their minds much of the time. But they describe this as being just like having the radio on in the background. They know it is there, and they know what's on the program if they want to tune in to it, but they can get on with the rest of their lives. So the issue is not learning how to switch thoughts off, but how best we can change the way we relate to them: seeing them as they are, simply, streams of thinking, events in the mind, rather than getting lost in them. So when the mind wanders, the instruction is to acknowledge that it has wandered, note where it went, then gently return attention to the breath or body. The positive thing about this practice is that wherever your mind may be, you can always start again in the next moment. The essence of mindfulness is the willingness to begin over and over and over again.

One of the core skills in mindfulness practice is to disengage from old habits of mind. The body scan provides an opportunity to do this gracefully and gently. It can be seen as a practice of holding momentary experience in awareness and then letting go. That is easy to say. It turns out to be less easy in practice. The practice requires a deliberate decision: to bring the mind intentionally to each region, breathing into and out from it for a few moments, before (again, intentionally) moving the attention on to the next region of the body.

PRACTICE IN THE REAL WORLD

The first time that participants report on their homework practice always brings up a variety of responses. These emerge from both the discussion and the review of what participants have written in the diaries they keep on a day-to-day basis. Let us look at some examples of common reactions to doing the body scan practice during the week.

"I Couldn't Find Time to Do the Homework"

In each class, some participants report that they have simply not been able to do the homework, or have only practiced sporadically. Should we let such difficulties pass? Given the central role of homework in the program, it turns out to be more helpful to be explicit when this occurs, to let people know that the lack of homework will likely affect how much they will get out of the program, but without being critical of them. The task is to use occasions when participants have difficulty doing the homework as an opportunity to bring curiosity to bear upon what is going on. The participant's task for the next week is to bring an inquiring mind to the difficulty of finding time for the homework as it occurs. We find that this approach is more likely to help participants keep the door open to taking a second look at the problem, to bring awareness to the thoughts and feelings that might be blocking homework activity, and to note what is found.

"I Got Utterly Bored," "I Was So Irritated with the Tape"

These are some of the most compelling types of reactions because they undermine the very motivation to continue with the practice. In class, the instructor, typically, would deal with this feedback matter-of-factly, in an empathetic and accepting way, yet not surrendering the importance of practicing as if participants' lives depended on it. Such experiences can provide opportunities to work with negative emotions. In this way, the instructor embodies a way of relating to the difficulties that may be novel to participants and quite different from their usual ways of handling these feeling states. Responding to negative thoughts or feelings by being genuinely curious and accepting them as one's experience in the moment also provides a compelling first example of a stance toward negative emotions that is a recurring theme in MBCT. Asking questions about the feelings ("At what point did they arise? Were they constant or fluctuating? How long did they last? Did you notice if other thoughts, feelings, and bodily reactions were drawn in to the picture?" and so on) assists in getting a better "map of the terrain." These questions are not intended so much to "diagnose a problem" as to invoke a stance of nonjudgmental inquiry.

If participants ask, "What shall I do when I feel this way?," the spirit of inquiry can be maintained if the instructor asks what they have already done, and what happened next. Maintaining this curiosity is a more skillful approach than rushing to provide a "solution" based on the instructor's assumptions about a "best method." Often, participants have put tremendous effort into trying to control their bad feelings, and further suggestions (even, apparently, very wise ones) may simply feed their attitude that if only the right technique could be found, all their mood problems would be solved.

Does this mean that all suggestions are banned? No. Rather, the primary stance is to inquire and to question; suggestions, if they come, are borne of such inquiry. For example, one suggestion might be that participants simply choose to note any irritation or boredom as a state of mind. Then, once this has been registered, they can bring their awareness back to the part of the body on which they intended to focus. The invitation is that they use the suggestion to notice what happens when they employ this strategy during the body scan. This may provide for them an example of what happens when they intentionally disengage attention from processing to which the mind has been "automatically" pulled by emotion, and intentionally return it to a chosen object of awareness. Of course, this needs to be implemented over and over again during a period of formal practice. Putting suggestions in the context of inquiry allows participants to see them as part of furthering their discoveries about mind and body rather than attempts to fix their problems.

"It Was Great, I Fell Asleep,"
"I Enjoyed It Because I Was Finally Able to Relax,"
"It Didn't Do Anything for Me, I Just Fell Asleep"

If people find they are less tense, calmer, or if they fall asleep during the practice, they may believe that the body scan "worked" because it helped to induce a pleasant state, or that it "failed to work" because they did not comply with the instruction to be awake and aware. While the negative comments can be handled in the same way as the feelings of boredom we discussed earlier, it is sometimes surprisingly difficult to handle apparently positive comments. Being relaxed and enjoying the practice is often mixed with a feeling that this is the goal of the class. This is understandable from the point of view of participants wanting to get something out of the time and energy they put into this practice. Nevertheless, it will be important at some point to set these feelings in a wider context than mere relaxation:

> "OK, well, that's interesting, isn't it? And obviously we hope that this will eventually become a way of 'falling awake,' of learning how to relax into awareness. But keep in mind that the aim of the body scan is more to aid in the cultivation of awareness than an attempt simply to be relaxed. So we are not fixing any goals at all. It's simply a way of bringing attention to whatever is going on. Our bodies and minds are wonderful things, and if we don't get in the way, then we may sometimes find that they will just settle down into a sort of peaceful, gathered, relaxed state. And it sounds as if that's what has happened here. Just allowing the mind and the body to do those things, we may settle down into a relaxed state, or we may not. But the one thing to remember is that it's not a goal or an expectation. We are not sitting down with the intention of being relaxed by the end and checking to see if we are getting there or not. If you are tense throughout the whole thing and can bring your attention to the physical sensation in the body, then return to the part of the body you intended to focus on, that is it. You've done what you have to do."

The reasons for doing the body scan are more about finding a way to reestablish contact with the body, whether what comes up is pleasant or unpleasant. Looking to the body scan for its positive effects or benefits can get in the way of being with and acknowledging the wider range of reactions that can be revealed through this practice. Moreover, the practice of the body scan is aimed more at waking up than falling asleep. So if someone falls asleep, that is fine. But the instructor might also want to remind the person of the challenge to use it, perhaps, at another time of day, and to wake up to what is happening in his or her body.

"I Am Trying My Best and I Still Don't Think I Get It," "I Think I Need to Work Harder at It"

For most people, the experience of depression is aversive enough to motivate them to find ways of preventing its return. We fully expect that participants in MBCT will come to class with specific aims in mind, and many will be willing to work hard to reach these aims. Paradoxically, much of the emphasis in practices such as the body scan is on *not* working or striving for goals. Of that much we can be clear. But putting into words what it is, positively, that we are encouraging is much more difficult. Instead of striving for goals, we might tell people that the emphasis is on "being," "dropping into the experience of the moment," or "allowing things to be held in nonjudgmental awareness, exactly as they are in this moment." Some mindfulness teachers refer to "settling into" each moment. Each of these phrases attempts to capture in words a constellation of meanings and implications. All are trying their best to convey a sense that the practice involves letting go of the impulse to fix or change, to escape or make better, or to be somewhere else in this moment. One way of making sense of this is to recognize that striving and having a goal orientation may work well in certain areas of life. But with emotions, sometimes the best way to get from A to B is to really be at A.[71] The trick, of course, is to be at A in a way that is different from how one usually is there. But this, too, can sound like a riddle. Translated, it might mean that with emotions, sometimes the best way to change them is not to try to change them, but rather to bring awareness to them in order to see them more clearly. The final wrinkle here is that we must also beware that this is not just another subtle form of fixing.

Participants may be confused by the idea that "you don't need to get anywhere when you practice the Body Scan." After all, why bother doing this for 45 minutes a day, 6 days a week, if you get nothing out of it? An important point that easily gets lost in striving for outcomes is the fact that, with the body scan, our intention is to be fully present with the physical sensations in each moment. When looked at in this way, there is really nowhere else to go, so efforts to get anywhere else are misplaced and rob us of our power for learning and changing in profound ways.

One way of trying to achieve a balance between these competing demands in the mind (demands that are themselves normal and understandable) is to practice on a regular basis, but to do so without an attachment to specific goals or outcomes. This allows us to recognize that "progress" is possible in one's mindfulness practice and that a "particular" kind of effort is necessary in the practice of the body scan, but it is not a striving to achieve some special state.

"I Just Got Too Upset": Reconnecting with Avoided Emotion

Like many of us, people who have been depressed in the past often live in their heads rather than in their bodies. For one reason or another, they have found that it is "safer" to think *about* emotion (or anything else, for that matter) than to experience emotion in the body. In many patients, this strategy may have evolved as a general style for coping with emotion. For others, this retreat from the body to the mind began as a way to avoid intense emotion linked to specific, traumatic bodily experience. Physical or sexual abuse is an obvious example, but medical emergencies can also involve intense affect closely linked to bodily sensations. Although wholly understandable, the strategy of withdrawing attention from the body means that "processing" such emotional experiences remains uncompleted. Consequently, a continuing effort may be required to avoid having emotion-related bodily sensations enter awareness.

For such patients, intentionally reconnecting with awareness of bodily sensations, as the body scan practice requires, may be very difficult, or may even lead to experiences of being quite overwhelmed by previously avoided emotions. It is important in practice of the body scan for the instructor to be vigilant for hints in patients' feedback that they might be experiencing such difficulties. The instructor can then, very gently and sensitively, guide patients in how to relate skillfully to what might be quite frightening experiences, encouraging patients to walk the often fine line between, on the one hand, retreating entirely from bodily awareness, and, on the other, being "blown away" by the intensity of their experience. Intentionally returning awareness to the body scan instructions, and then following them by focusing on the specified region of the body, as best they can, provides patients with a way to "steady" themselves, while still remaining connected to bodily experience.

Although difficult, the effects of reconnecting with the body in this way can often be dramatically healing, allowing completion of the unfinished work of emotional processing. Listen to how one patient described this experience, looking backward from the perspective of Session 7:

> "I was quite alarmed when I started doing the body scan in the first couple of weeks. It was as if all my past was coming back to haunt me. I got very, very upset.
>
> "Now, I don't feel half as bad. I don't feel so stirred up about it all. I don't know where, but it's all been filed away now, and it's all very much neater and everything. I wish I knew then what I know now, and I might have been a bit more ready for it. It quite worried me that it all happened in the first couple of weeks, and I thought, 'Gosh, you know, it's just going to get worse and worse.' But it actually got better."

"My Mind Wouldn't Stay Still"

Many participants find that when they attempt formal or informal practice, some thought or feeling gets in the way. They may start to experience an inner monologue that runs something like the following:

"What's the point of doing this?"

"It didn't make me feel any better yesterday."

"This is too hard for me."

"I can't see what this has to do with my problems."

"I need more time in my life and this is just wasting time."

One response to this is simply to repeat the message that count-less people who have been through this before give to the beginner: "Just do it!" But side by side with that message, important though it is, it is essential to give participants some experience of recognizing the power of thoughts and interpretations in shaping feelings and behavior.

Let us take the example of two participants, whom we'll call Mary and Bob. Mary brought up the unanticipated obstacle of trying to find 45 minutes of free time. This prompted a whole series of thoughts. She wondered what this said about her. Was it simply that she was too busy, or did it mean that she was too concerned with making time for others, leaving little time for herself? We talked in the class about what her original intention had been: What had got in the way of it, and what other options might there be for her? These options could be explored as experiments during the next week.

Bob was able to find the time to practice but was unable to find a place that was quiet or private enough. In discussion in the class, we talked about whether his expectations about needing the "right" type of setting were getting in the way. In cases where it was not possible to have total quiet or privacy, we stressed that whatever space is cho-sen for practice is designed as much by our intention as by its physi-cal characteristics. Bob decided that he would try an experiment. He would continue to meditate upstairs, despite the fact that the chil-dren would be running and playing downstairs, with all the un-wanted noise, and rather than see this as a distraction, he would ex-plore how to work with the noise during the practice.

Both of the difficulties brought up by Mary and Bob can also represent an opportunity: They may allow people to observe the thoughts or feelings to which they give rise. This type of observation by participants leads naturally to further exploration of the power that thoughts can have over feelings and behavior. With this in mind, we move to the next exercise, taken from standard cognitive therapy practice.

THOUGHTS AND FEELINGS

Interpretation of events plays a large role in determining moods. Understanding the extent of this can be very helpful for many people in overcoming barriers in practice and in daily life. The link between thoughts and feelings is a basic premise of the cognitive model of emotional disorders, and by making it explicit, we aim to offer participants an additional rationale for the effort being asked of them throughout the program. Of course, one could opt simply to tell people about the connection, but using examples gives people the opportunity for a different sort of learning that connects more strongly to day-to-day experience and therefore has a greater chance of generalizing to everyday life.

Once people have settled into a comfortable position, we ask them to close their eyes and imagine the following scenario:

> "You are walking down the street, and on the other side of the street you see somebody you know. You smile and wave. The person just doesn't seem to notice and walks by."

We then invite participants to become aware of what is going through their minds, including any thoughts, feelings, or bodily sensations they might have. When participants open their eyes, we invite them to describe any feelings or bodily sensations they experienced and any thoughts or images that went through their minds. We list these reactions to the scenario on the board, patient by patient.

Some typical examples of responses are "I was upset (*feeling*) at them for not acknowledging me" (*thought*), "If you want to be stuck up, be stuck up" (*thought"*), "Fine, if that's how you feel, I don't care" (*feeling*), "You must have seen me. Do what you want" (*thought*), "I felt quite isolated" (*feeling*), "Nobody likes me" (*thought*), "I would be going over this in my head for quite some time. My thinking would be really negative, and every time I went down one branch, there would be three to five negative thoughts coming off that" (*description of thought processes—the actual feelings and thoughts*).

Note how the same situation elicits many different thoughts and interpretations, hence, many different feelings. This observation can then be used as the basis for discussion of how emotional reactions are often the product of our interpretations of events.

CONNECTING THE COGNITIVE MODEL OF DEPRESSION WITH THE THOUGHTS AND FEELINGS EXERCISE

The main message to draw from this exercise is *that our emotions are consequences of a situation plus an interpretation.* This is the basic ABC model of emotional distress. So often we find ourselves in a situation (A) and end up with a feeling (C). Normally, these are the things of which we are most aware. Often, we are not aware of a thought (B) that links them. It is as if there is this stream of thoughts present all the time, just under the surface, of which we are not aware. These thoughts are often not very obvious, particularly when we are not severely depressed, but they actually determine which emotion we feel, and how strongly we feel it.

In the approach taken in MBCT, dealing with and responding skillfully to this type of inner monologue is easier if it is spotted early enough. However, spotting it early is difficult, because it can occur quite automatically and overtake us, without our quite knowing what has happened. One minute we are thinking about the friend not noticing us; the next moment, we feel alone. Because of this, it is important to learn to see these automatic thoughts clearly for what they are. By bringing them to awareness, we have greater ability not to be carried away by the cascade of our emotions, and as in the raisin exercise, we may notice new things about our thoughts and feelings that we had not seen before. Note again that our investigations of these processes are borne out of curiosity rather than driven by problem solving.

At least two other themes emerge from discussion of this exercise. First, by looking at the variety of interpretations within the class itself, it is easy to see that our *interpretation of events* (and the feelings they evoke) reflect what we bring to them as much as the "objective" situation does.

> "One thing to notice is that all these different feelings come about because the same event is being given a lot of different interpretations. If you interpret the event as simply the other person not seeing you because of his or her own problems or from being preoccupied, then you feel sorry for the other person. If you interpret the event as being a rejection or a hostile gesture, then you get angry.
>
> "Now ask yourself which of these ways of thinking would be likely to come to mind if this happened when you were depressed. What thoughts would you be most likely to have if you were still depressed?
>
> "As this exercise shows, our thoughts are often powerfully determined by our present mood. The event itself is neutral in this particular case. All the action is on what you make of it. And what we are trying to do is to become more aware of these intervening thoughts."

The fact that interpretations of the same situation can vary, either over time (e.g., with mood) or from person to person, tells us that *thoughts are not facts*.

Second, *negative thinking is often a warning sign of oncoming depression*. For example, when we look at the list of reactions generated by the class, we can readily identify those statements that might be given by someone who is depressed. Most people agree that there is a strong connection between the types of interpretations listed and how depressed the person is. By comparing depressed thinking with nondepressed thinking we see just how powerfully distorting depression can be. Acknowledging this the next time these reactions pop into the mind enables us to "check in" with ourselves and see to what extent our thoughts and interpretations might have been distorted by depressed mood.

AWARENESS OF PLEASANT EVENTS

Becoming more fully aware of the way a situation is classified by the mind as "pleasant" or "unpleasant" and the extent to which our thoughts and moods color such interpretation may take some practice. Nor is it easy to be aware of all the effects that different situations and events (large and small) have on bodily sensations, feelings, and thoughts. With this in mind, we use an MBSR exercise for participants to complete as homework during the week. They are asked to be aware of at least one pleasant event that occurs each day (and preferably to become aware of it while it is occurring). The handouts include a calendar (see Pleasant Events Calendar, Handout 7.7) with spaces for them to write down, as closely as possible in time to any pleasant event, the thoughts, feelings, and body sensations that accompany the event. They are encouraged to write any thoughts down as if they were spoken out loud (in the words that actually came), using quotation marks, if that helps. Finally, they are asked to describe feelings and body sensations in as much detail as they can.

Why is it important to incorporate this exercise into an approach for persons who have been depressed? First, it brings mindful awareness to what may turn out to be a pivotal point in triggering rumination—the early and almost silent judgment about whether something is pleasant or unpleasant. Research from the laboratory of Russell Fazio[72] shows that, much of the time, we respond to incoming stimuli by classifying them as pleasant, unpleasant, or neutral. These are the trigger points for the mind to wander, and the purpose of this exercise is to make people aware of these pivotal moments. Bringing mindful awareness to bear at these moments may allow people to experience and appreciate the moment simply as it is, without adding further thoughts, for example, wishing it would go on for ever, or wondering why it does not happen more often.

Second, the exercise can help people notice what (even slightly) positive things may be occurring in their daily lives. Although it appears to resemble the pleasant events scheduling that is part of some structured treatments for acute depression, at this point in MBCT, the aim is not to increase the number of pleasant events but simply to become more aware of those that may already be there.

Third, the exercise may allow people to become more aware of the thoughts, feelings, and bodily sensations that accompany such pleasant experiences. The emphasis on awareness of physical sensations is not a prominent feature in cognitive therapy, but we included it because bodily sensations that accompany pleasant and unpleasant experiences can be a sensitive barometer of a person's affective state. In this way, such sensations can provide a signature or readout, in the body, of how a person is feeling from moment to moment.

Fourth, it is a nonthreatening way of introducing the practice of mindfulness, since the object at first is not any particular thought or emotion but rather a way in which thoughts and emotions can be recognized in novel and therefore potentially useful ways.

Together with the other homework assignments set for the following week (further formal practice using the body scan, bringing mindful awareness to another routine activity each day; see participant handouts for details), the aim is to link awareness of the body to awareness of the body's reactions and responses to everyday events.

ENDING THE CLASS: SITTING WITH THE BREATH

At this point, there needs to be a transition from the body scan, in which the attention is moved to various parts of the body, to a form of meditation in which the attention is kept on a single focus. We therefore follow the example of the Stress Reduction Clinic by finishing Session 2 with a brief sitting meditation, lasting 10 minutes, with awareness of breathing as the primary object of attention. The intention is to introduce the idea that to be better able to respond to old mental habits, we need to recognize them and have a way of releasing ourselves from their automatic grip. An important step is to practice paying attention to a single focus, in this case, the breathing, and to allow other distractions, such as thoughts, feelings, and sensations, to come and go in our minds without controlling attention.

Participants start simply by focusing attention on their breathing and then seeing what happens as they try and keep that focus. We ask participants to choose a comfortable posture that embodies a feeling of dignity and alertness. After a moment, we ask people to bring their attention to the breathing. The particular focus here involves paying close attention to the physical sensations of breathing: to be fully aware of each inbreath for its full duration and each outbreath for its full duration. As is bound to happen, the mind will eventually drift to other concerns. Every time people notice that their minds have wandered off the breathing, the instruction is to note what took it away and then gently escort the attention back to the sensation of the breath coming in and out. As often as the mind wanders from the breath, the task remains the same: simply to bring the mind back to the breath each time, no matter what has preoccupied it.

As Session 2 draws to a close, note the implicit message that ends it, an idea to which we returned again and again: It is just as valuable to become aware that the mind has wandered and to bring it back, as to remain fixed on the chosen object of attention (in this case, the breathing). This is all part of learning how to pay attention in this new way: on purpose, in each moment, and without judgment.

⊗

Summary of Session 2: Dealing with Barriers

Our aim in this program is to be more aware, more often. A powerful influence taking us away from being "fully present" in each moment is our automatic tendency to judge our experience as being not quite right in some way—that it is not what should be happening, not good enough, or not what we expected or wanted. These judgments can lead to sequences of thoughts about blame, what needs to be changed, or how things could or should be different. Often, these thoughts will take us, quite automatically, down some fairly well-worn paths in our minds. In this way, we may lose awareness of the moment, and also the freedom to *choose* what, if any, action needs to be taken.

We can regain our freedom if, as a first step, we simply acknowledge the actuality of our situation, without immediately being hooked into automatic tendencies to judge, fix, or want things to be other than they are. The body scan exercise provides an opportunity to practice simply bringing an interested and friendly awareness to the way things are in each moment, without having to do anything to change things. There is no goal to be achieved other than to bring awareness to bear as the instructions suggest—specifically, achieving some special state of relaxation is *not* a goal of the exercise.

HANDOUT 7.2

Tips for the Body Scan

1. Regardless of what happens (e.g., if you fall asleep, lose concentration, keep thinking of other things or focusing on the wrong bit of body, or not feeling anything), just do it! These are your experiences in the moment. Just be aware of them.

2. If your mind is wandering a lot, simply note the thoughts (as passing events) and then bring the mind gently back to the body scan.

3. Let go of ideas of "success," "failure," "doing it really well," or "trying to purify the body." This is not a competition. It is not a skill for which you need to strive. The only discipline involved is regular and frequent practice. Just do it with an attitude of openness and curiosity.

4. Let go of any expectations about what the body scan will do for you: Imagine it as a seed you have planted. The more you poke around and interfere, the less it will be able to develop. So with the body scan, just give it the right conditions—peace and quiet, regular and frequent practice. That is all. The more you try to influence what it will do for you, the less it will do.

5. Try approaching your experience in each moment with the attitude: "OK, that's just the way things are right now." If you try to fight off unpleasant thoughts, feelings, or body sensations, the upsetting feelings will only distract you from doing anything else. Be aware, be nonstriving, be in the moment, accept things as they are. Just do it.

---

1. Settle into a comfortable sitting position, either on a straight-backed chair or on a soft surface on the floor, with your buttocks supported by cushions or a low stool. If you use a chair, it is very helpful to sit away from the back of the chair, so that your spine is self supporting. If you sit on the floor, it is helpful if your knees actually touch the floor; experiment with the height of the cushions or stool until you feel comfortably and firmly supported.

2. Allow your back to adopt an erect, dignified, and comfortable posture. If sitting on a chair, place your feet flat on the floor, with your legs uncrossed. Gently close your eyes.

3. Bring your awareness to the level of physical sensations by focusing your attention on the sensations of touch and pressure in your body where it makes contact with the floor and whatever you are sitting on. Spend a minute or two exploring these sensations, just as in the body scan.

4. Now bring your awareness to the changing patterns of physical sensations in the lower abdomen as the breath moves in and out of your body. (When you first try this practice, it may be helpful to place your hand on your lower abdomen and become aware of the changing pattern of sensations where your hand makes contact with your abdomen. Having "tuned in" to the physical sensations in this area in this way, you can remove your hand and continue to focus on the sensations in the abdominal wall.)

5. Focus your awareness on the sensations of slight stretching as the abdominal wall rises with each inbreath, and of gentle deflation as it falls with each outbreath. As best you can, follow with your awareness the changing physical sensations in the lower abdomen all the way through as the breath enters your body on the inbreath and all the way through as the breath leaves your body on the outbreath, perhaps noticing the slight pauses between one inbreath and the following outbreath, and between one outbreath and the following inbreath.

(cont.)

6. There is no need to try to control the breathing in any way—simply let the breath breathe itself. As best you can, also bring this attitude of allowing to the rest of your experience. There is nothing to be fixed, no particular state to be achieved. As best you can, simply allow your experience to be your experience, without needing it to be other than it is.

7. Sooner or later (usually sooner), your mind will wander away from the focus on the breath in the lower abdomen to thoughts, planning, daydreams, drifting along—whatever. This is perfectly OK—it's simply what minds do. It is not a mistake or a failure. When you notice that your awareness is no longer on the breath, gently congratulate yourself—you have come back and are once more aware of your experience! You may want to acknowledge briefly where the mind has been ("Ah, there's thinking"). Then, gently escort the awareness back to a focus on the changing pattern of physical sensations in the lower abdomen, renewing the intention to pay attention to the ongoing inbreath or outbreath, whichever you find.

8. However often you notice that the mind has wandered (and this will quite likely happen over and over and over again), as best you can, congratulate yourself each time on reconnecting with your experience in the moment, gently escorting the attention back to the breath, and simply resume following in awareness the changing pattern of physical sensations that come with each inbreath and outbreath.

9. As best you can, bring a quality of kindliness to your awareness, perhaps seeing the repeated wanderings of the mind as opportunities to bring patience and gentle curiosity to your experience.

10. Continue with the practice for 15 minutes, or longer if you wish, perhaps reminding yourself from time to time that the intention is simply to be aware of your experience in each moment, as best you can, using the breath as an anchor to gently reconnect with the here and now each time you notice that your mind has wandered and is no longer down in the abdomen, following the breath.

⊗

The Breath

Breath is life. You could think of the breath as being like a thread or a chain that links and connects all the events of your life from birth, the beginning, to death, the end. The breath is always there every moment, moving by itself like a river.

Have you ever noticed how the breath changes with our moods—short and shallow when we're tense or angry, faster when we're excited, slow and full when we're happy, and almost disappearing when we're afraid? It's there with us all the time. It can be used as a tool, like an anchor, to bring stability to the body and mind when we deliberately choose to become aware of it. We can tune into it at any moment during everyday life.

Mostly, we're not in touch with our breathing—it's just there, forgotten. So one of the first things we do in mindfulness-based stress reduction is to get in touch with it. We notice how the breath changes with our moods, our thoughts, our body movements. We don't have to control the breath. Just notice it and get to know it, like a friend. All that is necessary is to observe, watch, and feel the breath with a sense of interest, in a relaxed manner.

With practice, we become more aware of our breathing. We can use it to direct our awareness to different aspects of our lives. For example, to relax tense muscles, or focus on a situation that requires attention. Breath can also be used to help deal with pain, anger, relationships or the stress of daily life. During this program, we will be exploring this in great detail.

From Karen Ryder, Instructor, Stress Reduction Clinic, University of Massachusetts Medical Center (personal communication). Reprinted by permission.

⊗

Homework for Week Following Session 2

1. Use the Body Scan Tape for 6 days and record your reactions on the record form.

2. At different times, practice 10–15 minutes' mindfulness of breathing for 6 days. Being with your breath in this way each day provides an opportunity to become aware of what it feels like to be connected and present in the moment without having to *do* anything.

3. Complete Handout 7.7, the Pleasant Events Calendar (one entry per day). Use this as an opportunity to become really aware of the thoughts, feelings, and body sensations around one pleasant event each day. Notice and record, as soon as you can, *in detail* (e.g., use the actual words or images in which the thoughts came) the precise nature and location of bodily sensations.

4. Choose a new routine activity to be especially mindful of (e.g., brushing your teeth, washing dishes, taking a shower, taking out garbage, reading to kids, shopping, eating).

Homework Record Form—Session 2

Name: _____

Record on the Homework Record Form each time you practice. Also, make a note of anything that comes up in the homework, so that we can talk about it at the next meeting.

Day/date	Practice (Yes/No)	Comments
Wednesday Date:	Tape: Breath:	
Thursday Date:	Tape: Breath:	
Friday Date:	Tape: Breath:	
Saturday Date:	Tape: Breath:	
Sunday Date:	Tape: Breath:	
Monday Date:	Tape: Breath:	
Tuesday Date:	Tape: Breath:	
Wednesday Date:	Tape: Breath:	

⊗

Pleasant Events Calendar

Name: _____

Be aware of a pleasant event *at the time it is happening*. Use the following questions to focus your awareness on the details of the experience as it is happening. Write it down later.

What was the experience?	Were you aware of the pleasant feelings while the event was happening?	How did your body feel, in detail, during this experience?	What moods, feelings, and thoughts accompanied this event?	What thoughts are in your mind now as you write this down?
Example: Heading home at the end of my shift—stopping, hearing a bird sing.	*Yes.*	*Lightness across the face, aware of shoulders dropping, uplift of corners of mouth.*	*Relief, pleasure, "That's good," "How lovely (the bird)," "It's so nice to be outside."*	*It was such a small thing but I'm glad I noticed it.*
Monday				
Tuesday				

(cont.)

155

Pleasant Events Calendar (p. 2 of 2)

Wednesday			
Thursday			
Friday			
Saturday			
Sunday			

CHAPTER 8

⍟

Mindfulness of the Breath
SESSION 3

How do we pick up our coffee cup from a tray full of cups? That is, how do we not only recognize it as ours but also successfully "navigate" around other cups and pick up our own, without knocking everything over? Research into the cognitive processes that underlie reaching for objects finds that the brain carries out a delicate balancing act between excitation of the object that is to be selected and inhibition (damping down) of the objects that are not to be selected. This balancing act has been finely tuned throughout our evolutionary history. Animals whose brains could not carry out the process would soon die: They would miss the branch for which they were leaping or the prey on which they were pouncing.

Because the skill of reaching seems so basic, when computer-assisted robots were first developed, it was assumed that they could easily be taught how to recognize and pick up a cup from among a group of cups. By contrast, it was assumed that teaching a computer to play a complex game such as chess would take much longer. It turned out to be the other way around. The chess-playing computer turned out to be relatively unproblematic: It simply demands a huge memory and fast consideration of millions of possibilities. But the computer that can do what a 3-year-old can do, in terms of recognizing a cup and picking it up without accident from among a group of similar cups, has taken much longer to develop. The computational power needed by the brain to carry out even the simple action of picking up a cup is immense, yet, even for a small child, it soon happens automatically, without awareness. Evolution gave us these skills long before consciousness developed. Perhaps because we have been exercising these skills since early childhood, we take them for granted and overvalue the more complex, "intellectually demanding" skills. Such intellectual skills are good for solving certain sorts of problems. They are particularly helpful when careful analysis is required. For example, the current situation (A) is compared with the desired state (B), and the various possibilities of getting from A to B are considered.

It is natural for us to believe that such intellectual problem solving might also help to solve our emotional problems. It seems plausible enough. The goal is clear: to escape or avoid unhappiness on the one hand, and to achieve happiness on the other. The problem is that this drive for happiness creates rumination: patterns of thinking, feeling, and behavior that are unhelpful because they simply circle round, and round without producing a resolution. Ruminating about a problem feels as if it should bring a solution, but as Susan Nolen-Hoeksema has found (see Chapter 2), such ruminations can often exacerbate the situation.

Such constant monitoring of how we fare against the standards of happiness we have set for ourselves turns out to be very unhelpful. To cope with waking in the morning feeling bad is difficult enough, but we often compound the mood by matching it against some standard, better mood. Soon, we find the results of this "matching" process going through our minds: "Why am I feeling this way? I am usually more cheerful than this; I shouldn't feel this way." We are soon trapped in verbal, problem-solving techniques—imagining that as in playing chess, if we could find just the right move, we would win the game.

We mention this now because we find that, following initial enthusiasm, Session 3 often brings up, with full force, the barriers (and other problems) we alluded to in Session 2. In the first two sessions, we have begun to explore how being mindful can help in stepping

out of the types of habitual patterns of thinking that can quickly escalate to cause depression. Whether people are able to see the relevance of it for their own lives and their own problems, they are generally prepared to suspend judgment. By Session 3, it becomes
clearer that this practice is not going to provide a ready-made set of
solutions to their problems, and frustration can set in. There may be
many sources for such frustration, but one common source is the feeling that our clever problem-solving abilities should be able to sort
out all our problems. The feeling is very compelling and cannot be
easily switched off. In fact, it is unlikely that persons would volun-
tarily give up their old ways of trying to deal with their problems by
ruminating about them unless they had sampled an alternative approach.

Yet the mindfulness-based approach does not involve just another, more clever problem-solving technique. Rather, it involves a
different mode: a way of "being with" problems that allows the person to let go of the need to solve them instantly. In stepping back
from the tendency to want instant solutions, we are inviting people to
see how much behavior is driven by avoidance of unpleasantness and
attachment to pleasantness. Simply being aware of the difficulty, and
holding it in awareness, can provide a time-out from getting caught
in old mental routines. Mindfulness practice involves sampling the
"being" mode, in which we are invited to let go of our usual striving
and goal orientation.

In the process of letting go, we may, ironically, be able to become
more open to seeing more clearly what is a skillful next step to be
taken when a problem arises. This involves allowing the mind to find
a balance between calmness and wakefulness. All the practices
learned during the classes and practiced at home are in the service of
sampling this new approach; many of the problems that arise in the
practice can be traced to the understandable difficulty in trusting that
this new way of approaching problems will be sufficient.

The next step in the program therefore involves developing
mindfulness of the breath, so that people can deepen their use of
breathing as an anchor to gather and steady themselves, while at the
same time being open to their experience, whatever it is. Once again,
the challenge is to find ways that people in the class can sample this

different approach. Recall that one of the attractions of the mindfulness approach in reducing risk of recurrence in those who are not currently depressed is that it can be applied to any experience, whether positive or negative, important or trivial. That is why we emphasize the combination of formal practice (such as the body scan) with informal practice (such as bringing awareness to a routine activity such as eating). If our task is to enable people to sample ways of looking at the world that are different from the "analytic" or "intellectual," then it is possible to use even the most basic sensations, such as seeing.

Consider the page you are reading right now. In order to read, you must see the marks on the page, analyze them as words and sentences, then fold together the sentences to understand the text as a whole. "Seeing" is most often simply what comes before such analysis in most of our daily lives. The way we "parse" the text happens so automatically, it is difficult to disentangle the processes. It also happens with objects and sounds in the world. Our attention naturally and automatically "parses" the world, categorizing and laying it out, ready to be acted upon by our intellect. One approach to offering a different way of being is therefore to take this most automatic of situations and renew our acquaintance with the sensations that go to make up the raw material of experience.

One way to do this is to start Session 3 with a simple, 5-minute "seeing" or "hearing" exercise. If there is a window in the room, we ask people to look outside, paying attention to sights as best they can, letting go of the categories they normally use to make sense of what they are looking at; rather than viewing elements of the scene as trees or cars, or whatever, we ask them simply to see them as patterns of color and shapes and movement. The instruction is that whenever participants become aware that they have started to think *about* what is being seen, they gently bring the attention back to simply seeing. If a window is not available, then we substitute a "hearing" meditation, asking people to listen to sounds in the room. The class is invited to bring attention to hearing, again, as best they can, letting go of the categories normally used to make sense of what is heard; instead of hearing a chair scraping or a person coughing, to hear the sounds as patterns of pitch, tone, and volume. Every time the mind wanders,

BOX 8.1

⊗

Theme and Curriculum for Session 3

THEME

With a greater awareness of how the mind can often be busy and scattered, learning to take awareness intentionally to the breath offers the possibility of being more focused and gathered.

AGENDA

- Five-minute "seeing" or "hearing" exercise.
- 30- to 40-minute Sitting Meditation (awareness of breath and body; what to do with intense physical sensations).
- Practice Review.
- Homework Review (including body scan, mindfulness of the breath and routine activity, and Pleasant Events Calendar).
- 3-Minute Breathing Space and review.
- Mindful Stretching and review.
- Mindful Walking and review.
- Unpleasant Events Calendar.
- Distribute Session 3 participant handouts.
- Homework assignment:
  Sitting Meditation Tape with stretches on days 1, 3, and 5.
  Yoga on Side 2 of Body Scan Tape on days 2, 4, and 6.
  Unpleasant Events Calendar (daily).
  3-Minute Breathing Space, three times daily.

PERSONAL PREPARATION AND PLANNING

- In addition to your personal preparation, remember to bring the audiotapes that combine mindful stretching and the sitting meditation.

PARTICIPANT HANDOUTS

Handout 8.1. Summary of Session 3: Mindfulness of the Breath.
Handout 8.2. The 3-Minute Breathing Space—Basic Instructions.
Handout 8.3. Homework for Week Following Session 3.
Handout 8.4. Homework Record Form—Session 3.
Handout 8.5. Unpleasant Events Calendar.

the attention is gently brought back just to hearing. In this way, we seek to make a transition from the "doing" mode in which people often arrive at the class, to the being mode, which is further explored in the mindfulness of the breath that immediately follows the focus on seeing or hearing.

THE SITTING MEDITATION
AS MINDFULNESS PRACTICE

For centuries, people have used breathing as a vehicle for meditation. Why should it be relevant to people who have been depressed in the past and remain vulnerable to becoming depressed again? Recall that in our analysis the escalation of negative thoughts in the face of mild states of negative mood was responsible for relapse and recurrence of depression. At times of potential relapse, an evaluation of something as positive or negative, particularly depressed mood itself, can set in motion a rumination ("Why do I not have more of this? Why do I have too much of that?"). Very soon, the mind is lost in thinking about the past or worrying about the future. Now, think about what the breath is and what it does.

First, it takes place in the present, so that focusing attention on it can help a person to let go of the past and the future. Second, it is always there, and therefore always available for focus as a marker of one's emotional state. Third, the very act of intentionally bringing awareness to the breath involves "taking up space" in the same limited capacity channel that has been filled with ruminative thought. So, although this is not the eventual aim, it can provide a temporary substitute for (or distraction from) the ruminative thinking. As alternative focuses of attention go, it is also useful because it is a "moving target" and requires some effort on the part of participants to maintain attention. Fourth, attention to the breath involves attending to something that is the opposite of goal orientation. It is not the participant's job to make the breath do its work. It simply does it. This attitude to the breath embodies a more general attitude toward the self and the world: that in one's emotional life, attention to the simple can be more effective than analysis of the complex. And because persons have breathed all their lives, it can link with many different situations, thereby giving it the potential to transform many situations. Finally, the simple act of registering that the mind has wandered, noting where it has gone, and returning to the breath involves just the sort of metacognitive monitoring—seeing thoughts as thoughts—that promotes the skills of decentering that will be needed to prevent the escalation of negative thought–affect spirals at times of potential relapse. Most importantly, such acts also provide repeated practice in intentionally disengaging from one mode of mind and engaging another—shifting mental gears from a mode that may increase rumination to one that emphasizes direct experience.

Before beginning the sitting practice, it is important that participants find a sitting posture that embodies, for them, a sense of calmness and dignity. Images of meditation in the media often bring to mind a person sitting cross-legged in a full lotus posture. In fact, the most important thing is to find a way of sitting that has comfort and stability. If this can be accomplished by sitting or kneeling on the floor, using a cushion or bench for support, or by sitting on a chair, then that is all that is required.

We use the same format as for the 10- to 15-minute sitting meditation introduced in Session 2. We begin by paying attention to posture, noting how the back should be upright but not stiff, aligned with the neck and head, the shoulders relaxed, and the chin tucked in a little. After a few moments, the instructor brings the focus of attention to the breath. This is now going to be the primary focus of awareness. The theme for this practice is clear and simple: *If your mind wanders, briefly notice what it is that took your mind away and then gently bring your attention back to your breathing, without giving yourself a hard time.* The instructions are repeated a number of times throughout the 30-minute sitting mediation, with various reminders to see whether the attention was on the breath at that very moment. Toward the end of the practice, participants are instructed to expand the awareness to the whole body (see Box 8.2).

The simplicity of this practice is important. Because it appears, on the face of it, to be so simple, it reveals all the more readily the dif-

BOX 8.2

⊗

Sitting Meditation:
Mindfulness of the Breath and Body

1. Practice mindfulness of the breath, as described earlier (p. 150), for 10–15 minutes.

2. When you feel reasonably settled on awareness of the breath, intentionally allow the awareness to expand around the breath to include, as well, a sense of physical sensations throughout the whole body. While still aware, in the background, of the movements of the breath in the lower abdomen, change your primary focus, so that you become aware of a sense of the body as a whole and of the changing patterns of sensation throughout the body. You may find that you get a sense of the movements of the breath throughout the body, as if the whole body were breathing.

3. If you choose, together with this wider sense of the body as a whole, and of the breath moving to and fro, include awareness of the more local, particular patterns of physical sensations that arise where the body makes contact with the floor, chair, cushion, or stool—the sensations of touch, pressure, or contact of the feet or knees with the floor; the buttocks with whatever supports them; the hands where they rest on the thighs, or on each other. As best you can, hold all these sensations, together with the sense of the breath and of the body as a whole, in a wider space of awareness of physical sensations.

4. The mind will wander repeatedly away from the breath and body sensations—this is natural, to be expected, and in no way a mistake or a failure. Whenever you notice that your awareness has drifted away from sensations in the body, you might want to congratulate yourself; you have "woken up." Gently note where your mind was ("thinking"), and kindly focus your attention back to your breathing and to a sense of your body as a whole.

5. As best you can, keep things simple, gently attending to the actuality of sensations throughout your body from one moment to the next.

6. As you sit, some sensations may be particularly intense, such as pains in the back or knees or shoulders, and you may find that awareness is repeatedly drawn to these sensations, and away from your intended focus on the breath or body as a whole. You may want

(cont.)

to use these times to experiment with intentionally bringing the focus of awareness into the region of intensity and, as best you can, explore with gentle and wise attention the detailed pattern of sensations there: What, precisely, do the sensations feel like? Where exactly are they? Do they vary over time or from one part of the region of intensity to another? Not so much thinking about it, as just feeling it, you may want to use the breath as a vehicle to carry awareness into such regions of intensity, "breathing in" to them, just as in the body scan.

7. Whenever you find yourself "carried away" from awareness in the moment by the intensity of physical sensations, or in any other way, reconnect with the here and now by refocusing awareness on the movements of the breath or on a sense of the body as a whole. Once you have gathered yourself in this way, allow the awareness to expand once more, so it includes a sense of sensations throughout the body.

ficulty that all of us have in putting aside the normal mode in which we operate. For people who have been depressed, the thoughts and feelings that come up may echo themes similar to the ruminations that would normally keep them vulnerable.

For example, people often link the practice they have just completed with their experience during the week and conclude that the practice is just too difficult, or that they are simply not up to the task:

P: I've got all the time in the world, really, to do it, but I only need one noise, and that takes it away instantly.

Note how this person believes that there is something she "has" that can be "taken away." The instructor asks for more information:

I: What happens when the noise comes?

The open-ended question is important, for the person's response reveals that behind the frustration with being distracted by noise is another thought:

P: I think that I am letting you down, and I know it sounds stupid, but . . . well, I feel that I'm not really contributing like I should.

We can see here the machinery of rumination clanking into action. A noise occurs. It distracts. There is frustration at "losing it," rapidly followed by another thought about letting the instructor down because the participant is not contributing as she should. How does she deal with this negative thought? By telling herself that she sounds stupid! Here is rumination laid bare: a thought–affect spiral with escalating attempts to deal with a negative thought by criticizing the self for having it. The instructor decides to stay with this for a moment:

I: Let's stay on this, if you don't mind, because it's really important: this business about letting me down and not doing it properly, and having a whole set of expectations about what should be going on here. Now this is absolutely the target that we need to look at, because our aim here is simply, as best we can, to relate to what is there. The job you have is not to achieve a particular standard, but to be aware, if you like, of the thoughts that are saying "I have got to do well"; " I am letting him down," and so on. As best you can, say "Ah, there go those 'standards' again." As best you can, see them as judgments. It's very easy just to get sucked into those things and not see them for what they are. They are just things in the mind.

P: I find that I just talk to myself. "Here I go again," you know?

I: So it's ever so easy to get sucked in.

Staying with one person's experience enables other participants to see connections with their own experience. The transcript of the session shows a succession of participants building on the experience of this person:

P2:   I'm pleased, because it has worried me.

P3:   Unless there is absolutely peace and quiet, I can't do it. I've only done the practice once.

Once again, there turn out to be more negative thoughts lurking just in the background. It is not simply the difficulty; it is the self-criticism that comes along with the difficulty that really seems to bring the person's mood down.

P: I am ashamed to have missed it, and I didn't want to come tonight. I failed this week.

Once this rumination starts, rather like the last participant, it does not stop with mild self-criticism about the practice but escalates rapidly, until it connects with a theme that may have been very familiar to the person for some time:

P: I think to myself, "I only work. I haven't got a family, I haven't really got a busy life. What's wrong with me? Why can't I fit in?"

At one time, we would have felt drawn into using standard cognitive therapy techniques at this point. This would have involved asking more about the effect of such a thought on mood, and other situations in which the thought occurs. We might then have done some thought answering: investigating why it might be true that she did not fit in, and why it might be false. We would have worked on some homework tasks that might have given more evidence for and against the idea that she did not fit in.

But what if, instead, we encouraged people simply to label these thoughts as "judgment" and then, as best they could, return to the focus on the breath? This is what the instructor did in this case:

"OK. Well, as best you can, just notice this as judgment, and just let it go. It comes from somewhere, and it's no friend of yours, but you know, just treat it as kindly as you can. 'Oh, hello, Mr. Judgment. Here you are again. Have a nice day!' And, as best you can just bring your mind back to where you intended it to be."

It turns out that using the practice to learn how to relate differently to negative thoughts proves to be one of the most helpful aspects of MBCT.

MIND WANDERING

To describe the sitting meditation as spending 30–40 minutes with the focus of attention on the breath is somewhat misleading. Most people at this stage in the program spend a good deal of time struggling to maintain their attentional focus as it is pulled off the breath by thoughts, feelings, bodily sensations, or external distractions.

An essential characteristic of this practice is that the aim is not really to prevent mind wandering, but to become more intimate with how one's mind behaves. One important practice in the early stages is systematically and repeatedly to bring the attention back from wherever it may have wandered to the primary object of the meditation. In this way, the practice always gives us the chance to begin again, in this moment, with this breath. A common instruction one hears is "If your mind wanders a hundred times, then simply bring it back a hundred times." This is what the practice is all about. The task is to accept those times when our minds have wandered and *gently* reconnect with our breathing. This allows us to sidestep the judgments and criticisms that may arise from believing that we are failing at it or not doing well enough at keeping our attention locked on the breath. Becoming aware of the feeling of "struggling to maintain awareness on the breath" is itself helpful. At this stage in the program, such struggling is seen as simply another feeling to become aware of, before gently bringing attention back to the breath.

In the discussion of participants' actual experiences with the sitting meditation, several themes are often raised. We present them here, with an accompanying link back to the themes of the program, but this is not intended to imply that an MBCT class becomes a question-and-answer session. Rather, the instructor seeks to explore with participants how each aspect of their experience can teach them something of their "internal geography": how they can learn to "read the map," seeing the connections among their thoughts, feelings, and body sensations. The difficulties reported in class are welcomed as a possible guide to what normally causes moods to deteriorate or prevents attention from being focused or quiet. By asking questions such as "What are you noticing about the feeling right now?", the discussion is grounded in moment-to-moment experience.

DEALING WITH THOUGHTS BY TRYING TO CONTROL THEM

"I don't know if anybody else has this problem. When my mind is completely going, I have been thinking of a thousand and one other things. It's very difficult to stop myself going into the future, thinking about things. I try to control it and maybe it works for 2 minutes but then I go off again."

Note how easily participants mishear the instructions for the practice. Look again at what has been said. "It's very difficult to *stop* myself. . . . I try to *control* it . . . maybe it *works* for 2 minutes but then. . . . " This approach is not about trying to suppress or control thoughts. If we were to try and push them away or squash them down, then they would be more likely to bounce back even more strongly. The practice involves developing a gentle, skillful way of simply becoming aware, of being able to recognize that "Here is thinking," and as best one can, let go of the thinking and focus back on the breath. It's not so much trying to control our thoughts as actually feeling comfortable with letting things be as they are, and then returning to the breath.

BEING CURIOUS* ABOUT WHERE THE MIND WANDERS TO

"It's really annoying sometimes. I find that I want my mind to stay in one place, but it just seems to go off and do what it wants to anyway."

*By the word "curious," we mean an attitude of alert interest or wise attention. This is, of course, different from the more obsessive "picking over" a problem or intellectually "thinking *about*" a problem.

Note the expression of a strong desire for a particular outcome. The person wants the mind to be a certain way, and it doesn't happen. Instead, our thoughts are rather more like monkeys running through trees; they are sort of "all over the place." We become aware of how the mind may have "jumped into some other tree" as soon as we can, and then we gently bring our attention back. This is how we come to develop a sense of intimacy with our mind states. It is much more flexible than wanting them to be a certain way. Instead, we just watch the mind as it moves. To bring a spirit of kindly interest or curiosity to what is happening is helpful, because it is obviously quite easy to get impatient and frustrated with ourselves.

SENSATIONS OF PHYSICAL DISCOMFORT

"I find that if I sit for too long, my legs start to fall asleep and my back aches. I don't really want to move because, I guess, it would disturb my concentration, but it gets too painful not to."

Physical discomfort is actually a good target on which to practice these developing skills because it can be so easily located in the field of awareness and is a strong sensation to bring to awareness. Obviously, the natural reaction to such discomfort is to tense or brace and push it away. Simply becoming aware of that tendency and bringing, as best we can, a friendly interest to it, and exploring it gently, provides a very useful practice. Another possibility would be to bring awareness to the sensation of discomfort itself. This requires a level of skill in sustaining nonreactive attention that may not be available to all participants at this stage of the program. For those who are ready, the instruction is to focus directly on the discomfort and pain (points 6 and 7 of Box 8.2). For others, the instruction is as follows: if the mind is pulled away to intense sensations, this is noted, and attention is returned to the breath, using the breath as an anchor to which to return again and again. Later in the program, participants will have the opportunity to learn further how to focus on the difficult and unwanted.

RECOGNIZING PATTERNS
OF AUTOMATIC THINKING

"What's wrong with me? Why can't I find the time to practice the meditation?"

The challenge in all this work is learning how to observe our experience in a friendly way, rather than identifying with it, resisting it, or rejecting it. As we said earlier in the example of the person who thought she did not fit in, one way to approach negative automatic thoughts is just to notice them as best we can, label them as "judgment," and simply let them go. The really difficult thing is simply to notice them, without criticizing oneself for having them. The thought, "I wish I did not have these thoughts about so-and-so," too easily turns into "I ought to be over this by now. I must be such a weak and immature person." The aim here is not to try and block them out. Instead, we practice being with them in a different way and letting go of the need to engage with them, answer them back, or reassure ourselves through denying their validity. We can be here, and so can our thoughts, but this does not mean we must be tied up with them in, our accustomed ways. Being more aware of how our attention moves around is an important ally in this process.

WHAT TO DO WHEN STRONG
EMOTIONS ARISE

"I often find myself identifying with my emotions, believing that they define my experience. Then I feel trapped and hopeless. How can I work with these feelings?"

We can work with emotions by holding the feeling mindfully in awareness, without having to act on it. To say to ourselves, " Oh, anger is here" rather than "I am really fed up with her for talking to me that way," or "Here is fear" rather than "I'm terrified of making a mess of this presentation" allows us to be with the emotion in a way that does not require us to identify with it completely. In time, we also learn that the feeling itself may constantly be changing shape; it can become stronger or lose intensity over short intervals. Some instructors picture the mind as being like a vast, clear sky. All our feelings, thoughts, and sensations are like the weather that passes through, without affecting the nature of the sky itself. The clouds, winds, snow, and rainbows come and go, but the sky is always simply itself, as it were, a "container" for these passing phenomena. We practice to let our minds be that sky, and to let all these mental and physical phenomena arise and vanish like the changing weather. In this way, our minds can remain balanced and centered, without getting swept away in the drama of every passing storm.

THE PLEASANT EVENTS CALENDAR

A common theme to emerge from the previous comments is the difficulty in dealing with negative thoughts, feelings, and body sensations. Of course, it is rare that people even make the distinction between these three aspects of mind–body phenomena. In order to make the distinctions, it is helpful to use the feedback on the Pleasant Events Calendar, which gives everyone the chance to reflect with each other on what happened when they tried to record such moments, and to record exactly the thoughts, emotions, and body sensations that occurred in the moments they describe. We find it is helpful to use a blackboard to record responses to this exercise, distinguishing between (and listing separately) the different elements that emerge: Was that a thought or a bodily sensation or an emotion?

One thing that often emerges first is how apparently trivial moments often contain elements and dimensions of which we are not aware. Second, the distinction between thoughts, emotions, and body sensations comes as a revelation to many participants. Such distinctions are so evident to psychologists and other health professionals that it is easy to overlook how they are not readily part of everyday experience. Third, the exercise reveals that some people find it particularly difficult to become aware of subtle body sensations. Whatever the reason, the fact that the body is sending signals to the brain all the time, signals that are generally ignored most of the time, is an important discovery. The fact that these body sensations can be used to recognize subtle changes in emotion proves very useful for many people.

GENERALIZING THE PRACTICE: THE 3-MINUTE BREATHING SPACE

It is not unusual for people who are coping with the demands of developing a formal meditative practice to forget about the need to incorporate this practice into their daily lives. Some "generalization practice" is important to link what is being learned to a larger range of different situations. Generalizing what is learned in formal practice is not easy. Of course, we have already given instructions on how to make mindfulness a routine activity (e.g., brushing teeth, feeding the cat, taking out the garbage). But we need to go further and bring small parts of the formal practice into daily life. We have developed a "minimeditation" for this purpose: the 3-Minute Breathing Space.

The exercise is influenced by cognitive therapy practice in that it is very explicit and structured, in this case in focusing on how to bring mindfulness into everyday life. First, we program the breathing space to occur three times a day at set times. Then we ask people not only to use it at the preprogrammed times, but also, when they feel they need it, for example, if they feel stressed (introduced in Session 4). The result is that the 3-Minute Breathing Space becomes an important vehicle for bringing formal meditation practice into daily life. People find, first, that they can use it to deal with problems directly, as they are developing. Second, they find that it is a way to pause, even in the midst of a hectic day, and reestablish contact with the present moment.

There are three basic steps to the exercise. The first involves stepping out of automatic pilot to ask "Where am I?" "What's going on?" The aim here is to recognize and acknowledge one's experience at the moment. The second step involves bringing the attention to the breath, gathering the scattered mind to focus on this single object—the breath. The third step is to expand the attention to include a sense of the breath and the body as a whole (see Box 8.3).

BOX 8.3

⊗

Breathing Space—Transcript

"The first thing we do with this practice, because it's brief and we want to come into the moment quickly, is to take a very definite posture . . . relaxed, dignified, back erect, but not stiff, letting our bodies express a sense of being present and awake.

"Now, closing your eyes, if that feels comfortable for you, the first step is being aware, really aware, of what is going on with you right now. Becoming aware of what is going through your mind; What thoughts are around? Here, again, as best you can, just noting the thoughts as mental events. . . . So we note them, and then we note the feelings that are around at the moment . . . in particular, turning toward any sense of discomfort or unpleasant feelings. So rather than try to push them away or shut them out, just acknowledge them, perhaps saying, "Ah, there you are, that's how it is right now." And similarly with sensations in the body. . . . Are there sensations of tension, of holding, or whatever? And again, awareness of them, simply noting them. OK, that's how it is right now.

"So, we've got a sense of what is going on right now. We've stepped out of automatic pilot. The second step is to collect our awareness by focusing on a single object—the movements of the breath. So now we really gather ourselves, focusing attention down there in the movements of the abdomen, the rise and fall of the breath . . . spending a minute or so to focus on the movement of the abdominal wall . . . moment by moment, breath by breath, as best we can. So that you know when the breath is moving in, and you know when the breath is moving out. Just binding your awareness to the pattern of movement down there . . . gathering yourself, using the anchor of the breath to really be present.

"And now as a third step, having gathered ourselves to some extent, we allow our awareness to expand. As well as being aware of the breath, we also include a sense of the body as a whole. So that we get this more spacious awareness. . . . A sense of the body as a whole, including any tightness or sensations related to holding in the shoulders, neck, back, or face . . . following the breath as if your whole body is breathing. Holding it all in this slightly softer . . . more spacious awareness.

"And then, when you are ready, just allowing your eyes to open.

"Any questions or comments about that?"

After the exercise, participants are asked for feedback. Sometimes such feedback continues themes that have been brought up earlier in the class. Other times, however, new themes come up. The following is an example in which the theme of length versus brevity came up:

P: My attention wandered, not at the beginning, but about 15 seconds after I was into it. And then I got it together again. Is that because you're aware that it's going to be short?

I: It may be. The idea of being aware for a single breath seems doable; the idea of being aware of your breath for half an hour seems an enormous task. But in reality, you know, you can simply take it breath by breath. It's like having an enormous pile of logs in front of you that you have to move. If you contemplate the whole pile, your heart sinks and your energy fails. But you know if you could just focus on the one you've got to do now, give your full attention to that, then take the next one, then it becomes doable.

Notice how this can link with the sense many people have that they often exhaust themselves by anticipating all the things they have got to do, not just for this day, but for the rest of the week and the next month. They carry a burden that doesn't need to be carried. Tuning into just this moment, and into what is before them right now, allows the energy to come through, to complete just this moment's task.

Scheduling another formal practice in a day, even one as short as 3 minutes, will not happen automatically. The class members are therefore given some time to break up into pairs to discuss how they plan to arrange for three occasions each day to practice the 3-Minute Breathing Space over the coming week.

THE BODY AS A WINDOW ON THE MIND

Many participants report that their practice is sometimes dominated by a struggle to maintain balance in the face of negative ruminations.

In time, of course, the aim is to find a way of relating differently toward such rumination. Disengaging attention from such habitual patterns of the mind in a way that does not simply suppress or shut them out is subtle and can take a lot of practice. We emphasize that if people find they tend to engage in a battle between one thought ("Why did she say that?") and another ("That's a stupid thought"), then they always have the option of paying attention to how the thoughts and feelings affect their bodies. Bodily awareness helps us sample a different "mode" of being. Bringing awareness to a sensation in the body changes the nature of the emotional experience and gives us more choice about how to respond to what is here now. If we are aware of reacting to something emotionally, then the body may tell us our relationship to these feelings.

Paying attention to the body provides another "place" from which to view things, a different vantage point for relating to thoughts. If we want to get a perspective on our thoughts and feelings, if we can actually "be in" our bodies, then, we've got a different place from which to stand and look at the thoughts and feelings, rather than just in our heads. Finally, as we observed in Session 1, the body is often part of the feedback loop that maintains depressed mood (e.g., muscle tension keeps us locked in the loop of anxiety; a wilting posture keeps us in the loop of depression). Intentionally bringing awareness to the body can have two additional effects. First, paying attention to sensations of which we may not have been aware can change the experience of these sensations themselves, just as with the experience of mindfully eating the raisin in Session 1. Second, bringing awareness to the body allows persons to choose to alter one of the components of the "mode of mind" that is keeping them locked into an emotional state—by intentionally altering their posture or facial expression.

In the first 2 weeks, the body scan has been used to help people become more aware of bodily sensations. The formal practice of sitting meditation also involves becoming aware of body states. However, many people find it easier to focus on the body if it is doing something: stretching or walking. We therefore assign both breath- and body-based mindfulness practice as homework following Session

3, varying the day-to-day tasks by combining a short mindful stretching exercise (10 minutes), followed by a formal sitting meditation (for 30 minutes) one day of the week, and, on alternate days, using yoga (for 40 minutes) as the formal meditation practice.

We practice the 10-minute series of stretches in the class. Even within this short practice, a number of issues arise. First, such practice makes it easy to notice contrasts. For example, the effort required to hold a posture and the release associated with returning to a neutral stance is substantial. Similarly, the tension in the muscles used in raising up the arms and the rest that comes from bringing the arms back down to one's sides is significant. The task is simply to pay attention to these contrasts and notice the sensations associated with each phase of the prescribed movements. Practicing this in class also gives us an opportunity to remind people to monitor the attitude with which they do the exercises. This, itself, becomes a discovery for some people:

P: The advice is to focus our attention on the muscles and the feeling as we're doing them, isn't it?

I: Yes, I'm glad you raised that, because the point of this is, of course, not physical strengthening. It's just another opportunity to become aware of the body, only it's a bit easier because the body is moving. . . . The spirit in which you do it is important. That's why the tape will say to do it slowly and attend to the particular sensations that you are focusing on. . . . And with the 45-minute yoga, be careful if you have any problems with your back. Be ever so gentle with that. As it says, honor the messages from your body. . . . It's a wonderful opportunity for letting go of standards. It is easy to start imposing standards on yourself and making it torture. Instead, it's that spirit of just doing it lightly rather than making it a performance.

This response illustrates the theme of striking the right balance between just how much effort is required to put into a stretch, and how much can be held back so as to avoid injuring oneself. We emphasize that the idea is not to hold a posture until it is painful. It is rather to move into and back from the point at which one is aware of these strong sensations, while keeping attention on the sensations themselves, as best one can. Noticing the sensations themselves, such as burning, trembling, or shaking, the task is to breathe with the sensations, letting the thoughts about what it means to feel these things just come and go in awareness. It is not unlike the sitting meditation, where we escort our attention back to the breath, but in this case, we just focus on sensation and let go of whatever else is there. The skill built by doing this with physical sensations comes into play later in the program, when a similar approach is used for mindfully moving into and out of painful emotions.

Participants discover that they derive a number of benefits from doing this work. First, the physical sensations associated with stretching, pulling, holding, balancing, and other demands enable some people to learn more about their bodies. Second, many participants discover that their bodies become more supple and responsive to day-to-day demands placed upon them, even though they have not set this as a goal. Third, it allows some people to learn to distinguish sensations in one part of the body from those in other parts of the body. The result is that, even if participants feel tension, such sensations are more likely to be confined to a single area rather than spreading throughout the body.

As with the formal sitting practice, the issue arises as to how this greater awareness of physical sensations in the body can be generalized to daily life. One possibility is to take a physical action that we use every day and slow it down, performing it mindfully, so that the action itself can act as a bridge between practice and daily life. This is what is done in mindful walking.

MINDFUL WALKING

Mindful walking takes the everyday activity of walking and uses it as a mindfulness practice to become more aware of bodily sensations (see Box 8.4). We walk, knowing that we are walking, feeling the walking.

BOX 8.4

⊗

Mindful Walking

1. Find a place where you can walk up and down, without feeling concerned about whether people can see you. It can be inside or outside.

2. Stand at one end of your walk, with your feet parallel to each other, about 4 to 6 inches apart, and your knees "unlocked," so that they can gently flex. Allow your arms to hang loosely by your sides, or hold your hands loosely together in front of your body. Direct your gaze, softly, straight ahead.

3. Bring the focus of your awareness to the bottoms of your feet, getting a direct sense of the physical sensations of the contact of the feet with the ground and the weight of your body transmitted through your legs and feet to the ground. You may find it helpful to flex your knees slightly a few times to get a clearer sense of the sensations in the feet and legs.

4. When you are ready, transfer the weight of the body into the right leg, noticing the changing pattern of physical sensations in the legs and feet as the left leg "empties" and the right leg takes over the support of the rest of the body.

5. With the left leg "empty," allow the left heel to rise slowly from the floor, noticing the sensations in the calf muscles as you do so, and continue, allowing the whole of the left foot to lift gently until only the toes are in contact with the floor. Aware of the physical sensations in the feet and legs, slowly lift the left foot, carefully move it forward, feeling the foot and leg as they move through the air, and place the heel on the floor. Allow the rest of the bottom of the left foot to make contact with the floor as you transfer the weight of the body into the left leg and foot, aware of the increasing physical sensations in the left leg and foot, and of the "emptying" of the right leg and the right heel leaving the floor.

6. With the weight fully transferred to the left leg, allow the rest of the right foot to lift, and move it slowly forward, aware of the changing patterns of physical sensations in the foot and leg as you do so. Focusing your attention on the right heel as it makes contact with the ground, transfer the weight of the body into the right foot as it is placed gently on the ground, aware of the shifting pattern of physical sensations in the two legs and feet.

(cont.)

Mindful Walking *(cont.)*

7. In this way, slowly move from one end of your walk to the other, aware particularly of the sensations in the bottoms of the feet and heels as they make contact with the floor, and of the sensations in the muscles of the legs as they swing forward.

8. At the end of your walk, turn slowly around, aware of and appreciating the complex pattern of movements through which the body changes direction, and continue walking.

9. Walk up and down in this way, being aware, as best you can, of physical sensations in the feet and legs, and of the contact of the feet with the floor. Keep your gaze directed softly ahead.

10. When you notice that the mind has wandered away from awareness of the sensations of walking, gently escort the focus of attention back to the sensations in the feet and legs, using the sensations as the feet contact the floor, in particular, as an "anchor" to reconnect with the present moment, just as you used the breath in the sitting meditation.

11. Continue to walk for 10 to 15 minutes, or longer if you wish.

12. To begin with, walk at a pace that is slower than usual, to give yourself a better chance to be fully aware of the sensations of walking. Once you feel comfortable walking slowly with awareness, you can experiment as well with walking at faster speeds, up to and beyond normal walking speed. If you are feeling particularly agitated, it may be helpful to begin walking fast, with awareness, and to slow down naturally as you settle.

13. As often as you can, bring the same kind of awareness that you cultivate in walking meditation to your normal, everyday, experiences of walking.

It has been described as "meditation in motion": being with each step, walking for its own sake, without any destination. As with other mindfulness practices in this program, we use the movements and sensations of walking to bring ourselves into the present. The focus is on maintaining moment-to-moment awareness of the sensations accompanying our movements, letting go of any thoughts or feelings about the sensations themselves. This seemingly simple exercise can be a powerful teacher of a core message in MBCT, because our bodies are more anchored in the here and now, while our minds all too easily ricochet between the past and future. This anchoring allows a greater sense of who we really are in the present moment.

The practice turns out to be especially useful for those who feel agitated and unable to settle. The physical sensation of walking, people comment, tends to enable them to feel more "grounded." To some extent, this can be generalized across all the mindfulness exercises: When the mind is agitated or a person feels pressured, it is easier to be mindful with a practice that involves physical movement than with one that does not.

RECORDING UNPLEASANT EVENTS

The theme of being present in the moment is picked up when people complete the second part of the Unpleasant Events Calendar as homework during the week. This time, they are asked to record unpleasant events. But the task is the same as for pleasant events: to notice as clearly as possible the thoughts, feelings, and bodily sensations associated with unpleasantness, no matter how fleeting or momentary the event in question may be. Of course, some situations may be long-lasting and intense, but the task remains to notice these aspects and record them in detail and as soon as possible, afterwards. When discussing the Pleasant Events Calendar in Session 2, we saw that focusing on bodily sensations allows people to identify an important signature of their emotion.

Gradually, in many various ways, a deeper message is communicated through these exercises: that bringing awareness to each situation, especially those in which we label things as good or bad, is the first step in learning to relate differently to them. This takes some courage and much practice. People can be discouraged because nothing seems to be happening. But despite the early skepticism that we ourselves felt when first using this approach, evidence from the classes we have taught has shown us that staying with the practice, rather than rushing for solutions, is justified. The picture that comes to mind is the bucket put underneath a slowly dripping tap. If you stare at the bucket, it is difficult to see any change at all in how full it is, but it nevertheless fills up. Our experience has been that when people are able to set aside their goals and simply practice day by day, they start to notice unexpected changes. Gradually, they discover, little by little, that the old way of tackling their moods by ruminating about them might not be the only way, that the old way of running their lives by shouting at themselves might be able to give way to a gentler way of living their lives.

⚯
Summary of Session 3: Mindfulness of the Breath

Focusing on the breath:

- Brings you back to this very moment—the *here and now*.

- Is always available as an anchor and *haven*, no matter where you are.

- Can actually change your experience by connecting you with a wider space and broader perspective from which to view things.

BASICS

It helps to adopt an erect and dignified posture, with your head, neck, and back aligned vertically—the physical counterpart of the inner attitudes of self-reliance, self-acceptance, patience, and alert attention that we are cultivating.

Practice on a chair or on the floor. If you use a chair, choose one that has a straight back and allows your feet to be flat on the floor. If at all possible, sit away from the back of the chair so that your spine is self supporting.

If you choose to sit on the floor, do so on a firm thick cushion (or a pillow folded over once or twice), which raises your buttocks off the floor 3 to 6 inches.

⊗

The 3-Minute Breathing Space—Basic Instructions

I. AWARENESS

Bring yourself into the present moment by deliberately adopting an erect and dignified posture. If possible, close your eyes. Then ask:

"What is my experience right now ... in thoughts ... in feelings ... and in bodily sensations?"

Acknowledge and register your experience, even if it is unwanted.

2. GATHERING

Then, gently redirect full attention to breathing, to each inbreath and to each outbreath as they follow, one after the other.

Your breath can function as an anchor to bring you into the present and help you tune into a state of awareness and stillness.

3. EXPANDING

Expand the field of your awareness around your breathing, so that it includes a sense of the body as a whole, your posture, and facial expression.

The breathing space provides a way to step out of automatic pilot mode and reconnect with the present moment.

The key skill in using MBCT is to maintain awareness in the moment. Nothing else.

Homework for Week Following Session 3

This week we are going to use two different tapes:

1. On Days 1, 3, and 5, use the Combined Breath Focus Tape and record your reactions on the Homework Record Form. This tape combines a few minutes of gentle stretching exercises and instructions for mindfulness of the breath and body.

2. On Days 2, 4 and 6, use the yoga instructions on Side 2 of the Body Scan Tape, and record your reactions on the Homework Record Form.

   The point of the stretches and yoga is to provide a direct way to connect with awareness of the body. The body is a place where emotions often get expressed, under the surface, and without our awareness. As such, it gives us an additional place from which to stand and look at our thoughts. If you have any back or other health difficulties that may cause problems, make your own decision as to which (if any) of these exercises to do.

3. Practice using the 3-Minute Breathing Space three times a day, at set times that you have decided in advance, and record each time by circling an R on the Homework Record Form.

4. Complete the Unpleasant Events Calendar (one entry per day)—use this as an opportunity to become really aware of the thoughts, feelings, and body sensations in one unpleasant event each day, *at the time that they are occurring.* Notice and record, as soon as you can, in detail (e.g., put the actual words or images in which thoughts came, and the precise nature and location of bodily sensations).

   What are the unpleasant events that "pull you off center" or "get you down" (no matter how big or small)?

⊗⊗

Homework Record Form—Session 3

Name: _____

Record on the Homework Record Form each time you practice. Also, make a note of anything that comes up in the homework, so that we can talk about it at the next meeting.

Day/date	Practice (Yes/No)	Comments
Wednesday Date:	Tape: R R R	
Thursday Date:	Tape: R R R	
Friday Date:	Tape: R R R	
Saturday Date:	Tape: R R R	
Sunday Date:	Tape: R R R	
Monday Date:	Tape: R R R	
Tuesday Date:	Tape: R R R	
Wednesday Date:	Tape: R R R	

⊗

Unpleasant Events Calendar

Name: _____

Be aware of an unpleasant event *at the time it is happening*. Use these questions to focus your awareness on the details of the experience as it is happening. Write it down later.

What was the experience?	Were you aware of the unpleasant feelings while the event was happening?	How did your body feel, in detail, during this experience?	What moods, feelings, and thoughts accompanied this event?	What thoughts are in your mind now as you write this down?
Example: *Waiting for the cable company to come out and fix our line. Realize that I am missing an important meeting at work.*	*Yes.*	*Temples throbbing, tightness in my neck and shoulders, pacing back and forth.*	*Angry, helpless. "Is this what they mean by service?" "They don't have to be responsible, they have a monopoly." "This is one meeting I didn't want to miss."*	*I hope I don't have to go through that again soon.*
Monday				
Tuesday				

(cont.)

Unpleasant Events Calendar (p. 2 of 2)

Wednesday				
Thursday				
Friday				
Saturday				
Sunday				

CHAPTER 9

℅

Staying Present

SESSION 4

People who have been depressed in the past often spend a great deal of time and energy making comparisons. Perhaps today they feel a little better than yesterday, but are they still feeling worse than last week? Did that person's frown mean he or she feels differently about me? Has he or she lost patience with me? Such people have often suffered many losses and disappointments, together with the sense of rejection and worthlessness that often comes from such events. Long afterwards, the mood of someone who has been depressed remains easily upset by reminders of these bad times. Even when depression is gone, people can feel cheated of the years that the depression has taken out of their lives. "Why didn't my doctor diagnose me earlier?," "I have lost the best years of my life!" There is a natural tendency to return to the past and sigh, "If only."

Mindfulness approaches are not about thought control or substituting positive for negative images of the past, present, or future. Rather, they encourage people to allow these feelings of disappointment and regret to be there. This is very different than how we commonly react to difficult or painful experiences, which is to find a way of reducing their impact on us. Distraction and denial are frequently used to shut out painful feelings. On the other hand, when a person worries or ruminates about his or her problems, although he or she seems to be addressing the difficulty, such rumination actually takes the person further away from a direct sense of what the difficulty is. This happens because the rumination involves a judgment about the experience, for example, "I don't want to feel like this." It involves concept-based thinking—*thinking about* the feelings rather than directly experiencing them. Such ruminative thinking then escalates into more highly charged feelings, adding further negative thoughts: "My parents never talked about it to me. Nobody ever talked about it to me." With time, it becomes difficult to separate the raw experience from the judgments about it.

These reactions of avoidance or preoccupation reflect a desire for things to be different than they actually are at the moment. It is as if we feel compelled to put effort into changing the current state of affairs into "how it should be," in order to avoid having to face the unpleasantness or disappointment of how it actually is. This strategy appears to succeed often enough to reinforce its use. With time, we come to rely on it to take care of things automatically. However, it also locks us into a particular way of coping with unpleasant experiences, leaving little room for change. If unsuccessful, rather than change strategy, individuals redouble their efforts to use the same sort of avoidance or rumination to deal with the problem.

A LIGHTNESS OF TOUCH

A core theme of this program is that the best way to prevent relapse is to act on the basis of staying present with what is unpleasant in our experience. Why is this important? It allows the process to unfold, lets the inherent "wisdom" of the mind deal with the difficulty, and allows more effective solutions to suggest themselves. The idea of "inherent wisdom" can seem strange. However, it may be somewhat analogous to the experience of mathematicians who report that they have often struggled to find a solution to a puzzle, only to find that the answer comes, as if from nowhere, once they have given up thinking about it. Similarly, people report that when they practice mindfulness, it can feel as if a "process" is unfolding—as if their mind appears to find ways of handling difficulties that are wiser than their thinking. In particular, the practice of mindfulness allows people to suspend their habitual ways of relating to negative experience, often by stripping away judgment and expectation. If the old habits become less powerful, then it gradually becomes easier to take skillful action in response to difficult moods and situations, rather than simply to react automatically to them. Having a certain "lightness of touch" in our awareness of thoughts, feelings and body sensations evoked by events gives us the possibility of freeing ourselves from habitual, automatic ways of reacting.

But dealing with the negative is not easy. In the sitting meditation that people practiced during their homework, and which is practiced again at the start of Session 4, they may have become aware of negative thoughts and feelings. Simply returning to the breath is often very difficult under these circumstances. Once the experiences are judged to be unpleasant, it is natural to feel an aversion to such unpleasantness. The observation that such a reaction of aversion simply adds negativity to negativity may not seem to help things very much.

EXPLORING EXPERIENCE: ATTACHMENT AND AVERSION

At this point in the program, we remain with a relatively simple message (but a difficult practice!). The message at this stage is for people to explore ways of becoming more aware of their experience, whatever its quality, so that they might learn to respond mindfully rather than to react automatically. Two forms of automatic reaction to experience are of particular relevance. In the first, we react by wanting to hold on to the reaction (attachment), especially if something is judged to be pleasant; we don't allow ourselves to let go of an experience that we are having right now, or we wish to have other experiences that we are not having right now. In the second, we react by wanting the reaction to go away, by being angry with it (aversion), if something is

BOX 9.1

⊗

Theme and Curriculum for Session 4

THEME

The mind is most scattered when it tries to cling to some things and avoid/escape other things. Mindfulness offers a way of staying present by giving another place from which to view things: to help take a wider perspective and relate differently to experience.

AGENDA

- Five-minute "seeing" or "hearing" exercise.
- Forty-minute Sitting Meditation—awareness of breath, body, sounds, then thoughts.
- Practice Review.
- Homework Review (including Sitting Meditation/Yoga and 3-Minute Breathing Space).
- Defining the "territory" of depression: Automatic Thoughts Questionnaire and Diagnostic Criteria for Depression.
- 3-Minute Breathing Space + Review (read the poem "Wild Geese").
- Watch first half of *Healing from Within* videotape and discuss.
- 3-Minute Breathing Space and review.
- Hand out copies of *Full Catastrophe Living* to the class.
- Distribute Session 4 participant handouts.
- Homework assignment:
  Sitting Meditation Tape (Series 1, Tape 2), 6 out of 7 days.
  3-Minute Breathing Space—Regular (three times a day).
  3-Minute Breathing Space—Coping (whenever you notice unpleasant feelings).

PERSONAL PREPARATION AND PLANNING

- In addition to your personal preparation, remember to bring the *Healing from Within* video, copies of *Full Catastrophe Living*, the Series 1, Tape 2 audiotapes, and the poem "Wild Geese" to the class.

(cont.)

PARTICIPANT HANDOUTS

Handout 9.1. Summary of Session 4: Staying Present.
Handout 9.2. Homework for Week Following Session 4.
Handout 9.3. Homework Record Form—Session 4.
Handout 9.4. Staying Present.

---

judged to be unpleasant; we want to get rid of experiences that we are having right now, or we avoid future experiences that we do not want.

Because the theme of connecting to the present is examined in the sitting meditation, participants are asked to observe in the body these reactions of aversion or attachment that arise during the practice. They are invited to notice how such reactions are powerful competitors for attention and often take awareness away from the breath, moving the focus to other, seemingly vital thoughts or feelings. The practice of mindfulness can be a powerful ally, allowing us to notice when this has occurred and to regain the ability to choose where we wish to place our attention in this moment. Note, again, that the aim of the practice is not relaxation or even happiness. Rather, it is freedom from the tendency to get drawn into automatic reactions to pleasant and unpleasant thoughts, feelings, and events. But getting drawn into such thoughts and imaginings still happens—even for experienced meditators. The promise of mindfulness practice is not that such mind wandering will be prevented, but that a person will come to find it possible to extricate him- or herself from it in a nonjudgmental way when it does occur.

Although we have spoken about attachment and aversion, it is worth reminding ourselves that the skills necessary to deal with positive and negative issues can be learned on neutral or trivial thoughts and impulses that arise during the practice. To practice letting go of a thought about buying food for tonight's supper is an important contributor to the ability to free oneself from a rumination about whether one is capable of being a good parent to one's children. Such freedom is what "staying present" is all about.

People have used many ways to describe this "learning to stay present." Some refer to recovering a sense of balance. Others use the metaphor of a mountain that stays grounded on the surface of the earth despite the changing weather conditions around it. It is difficult to find the right words to express such a subtle but deep meaning. Simple descriptions and explanations may not capture a message that seems to require more than words. What is referred to here is an awareness not simply of thoughts or feelings, but of the entire mode of mind (including "felt senses" in the body and the tone of the voice in the head, not just what it is saying). So how can such messages best be conveyed? Poetry and parable may be needed to capture some of this subtlety (some examples of poems we used can be found in the participant handouts; for example, the instructor reads Mary Oliver's poem "Wild Geese" toward the end of the sitting practice during this session). But the importance of using the practice itself as a vehicle for learning cannot be overstated.

NARROWING AND WIDENING THE FOCUS OF ATTENTION

In this spirit, the class can once again start with a short "seeing" or "hearing" meditation as a way of "arriving/gathering" and coming into the present. Noticing just one feature in the field of sight or sound (such as a leaf on a tree or the sound of a car engine) and then spreading awareness out from it can be a powerful way of staying present: changing the mode of mind from "doing" to "being," from "problem solving" to "allowing." The instruction that, if new thoughts arise, we just let them go as best as we can and bring our minds back to what we see or hear reinforces this sense of letting go of the tendency to struggle with such thoughts.

In the same way, we have found that the move into the 30- to 40-minute sitting meditation provides another opportunity for learning. Once again, awareness of posture is the starting point. The aim is to feel stable and focus attention on just being with moment-to-moment experience. The instructions for the sitting meditation begin by focusing attention on the breath. If people notice their mind wandering, they simply note where it went, register the fact that it has gone, and then gently bring their attention back to the breath.

We find ourselves returning time and again to this gentleness when the mind has wandered, and gentleness in bringing attention back to the breath. Such gentleness is important because it conveys an attitude of caring to ourselves (whether an instructor or a participant) and to whatever the experience may be in the moment. Such gentleness is incompatible with the negative reactions that might occur at this point (e.g., "My mind has wandered again. I must be the worst meditator in the world," "Why did I ever think this practice would do anything for me?"). Instead, the practice is one of noticing, acknowledging, and then kindly and gently escorting the mind back to the breath and not just pulling it back abruptly.

In addition, it is important to remember that we are not trying to teach a method to control the breath. The task is simply to bring full care and attention to the actual physical sensations as the breath moves in and out of the body, allowing the breath to breathe itself. The breath is used as an anchor to reconnect to the present whenever the mind wanders.

The longer people sit, the more they will find themselves reacting to what they are doing. It is helpful at these times to remember that the easiest way to let go is simply to stop trying to make things different from how they are. The task remains just to note any thoughts and return to the breath. Practicing with the breath in this way will allow people to train their attention and observe the movement and patterns of the mind. With time they will learn to open awareness to whatever arises in the mind or body, and to use that as a focus.

This is encouraged at a certain point during the practice by *expanding* awareness to the *whole body* rather than simply to the breath. If the mind wanders, the task is the same: simply to note where it went and to bring attention back to the current focus—the sense of the body as a whole. We may become aware of sensations throughout the body, particularly noting any regions of intensity or discomfort. One way to work with this is intentionally bringing our awareness to those regions of intensity and breathing into them and breathing out from them (see Chapter 8, Box 8.2). The awareness is then extended beyond the body

BOX 9.2

⊗

Sitting Meditation:
Mindfulness of Sounds and Thoughts

1. Practice mindfulness of breath and body, as described earlier, until you feel reasonably settled.

2. Allow the focus of your awareness to shift from sensations in the body to hearing. Bring your attention to the ears and then allow the awareness to open and expand, so that there is a receptiveness to sounds as they arise, wherever they arise.

3. There is no need to go searching for sounds or listening for particular sounds. Instead, as best you can, simply open your mind so that it is receptive to awareness of sounds from all directions as they arise—sounds that are close, sounds that are far away, sounds that are in front, behind, to the side, above or below. Open to a whole space of sound around you. Be aware of obvious sounds and of more subtle sounds, aware of the space between sounds, aware of silence.

4. As best you can, be aware of sounds simply as sensations. When you find that you are thinking *about* the sounds, reconnect, as best you can, with direct awareness of their sensory qualities (patterns of pitch, timbre, loudness, and duration), rather than their meanings or implications.

5. Whenever you notice that your awareness is no longer focused on sounds in the moment, gently acknowledge where the mind had moved to, and then retune the awareness back to sounds as they arise and pass from one moment to the next.

6. Mindfulness of sound can be a very valuable practice on its own, as a way of expanding awareness and giving it a more open, spacious quality, whether or not the practice is preceded by awareness of sensations or followed, as here, by awareness of thoughts.

7. When you are ready, let go of awareness of sounds and refocus your attention, so that your objects of awareness are now thoughts as events in the mind. Just as, with sounds, you focused awareness on whatever sounds arose, noticing them arise, develop, and pass away, so now, as best you can, bring awareness to thoughts that arise in the mind in just the same way—noticing when thoughts arise, focusing awareness on them as they pass through the space of the mind and eventually disappear. There is no need to try to make thoughts come or go. Just let them arise naturally, in the same way that you related to sounds arising and passing away.

(cont.)

8. Some people find it helpful to bring awareness to thoughts in the mind in the same way that they might if the thoughts were projected on the screen at the cinema. You sit, watching the screen, waiting for a thought or image to arise. When it does, you pay attention to it so long as it is there "on the screen," and then you let it go as it passes away.

to include *sounds*, and then *thoughts*. Finally, the attention is allowed to focus on *whatever is most salient* in awareness, whether it be breathing, body sensations, sounds, or thoughts. The instructions here are simply to be aware of whatever comes up, "being with" whatever arises from moment to moment (see Box 9.2).

Notice the change during the practice from *focusing* attention (gathering) in the early stage to *expanding* attention in the later stage. It bears upon a distinction that meditation teachers draw between concentration aspects of meditation on the one hand, and mindfulness aspects on the other. Although discussing this distinction would take us too far beyond the scope of this session, it is worth pausing to reflect that the intention of the mindfulness approach is ultimately to allow people to become aware that there is a "larger space" in which thoughts may be held in awareness. Being able to hold a larger number of elements in experience at any one time is an important part of being sensitive to the wider context, and it contrasts with the narrower focus required at the outset to help "gather" oneself. The instructor reads Mary Oliver's poem "Wild Geese" toward the end of the sitting meditation (see Box 9.3).

During the time we were writing this book, a major U.K. millennium project, the Tate Modern Art Gallery, opened in London. A feature of the gallery upon which visitors commented was that it had large spaces, so that works of art could be seen from a wide perspective. It was different from the experience that people often report after visiting more conventional galleries, where too many people in too small a space means that a picture can only be seen from one angle, or from too close. By contrast, the new gallery gave viewers a sense of spaciousness.

BOX 9.3

⊗

"Wild Geese"

You do not have to be good.
You do not have to walk on your knees
for a hundred miles through the desert, repenting.
You only have to let the soft animal of your body
      love what it loves.
Tell me about despair, yours, and I will tell you mine.
Meanwhile the world goes on.
Meanwhile the sun and the clear pebbles of the rain
are moving across the landscapes,
over the prairies and the deep trees,
the mountains and the rivers.
Meanwhile the wild geese, high in the clear blue air,
are heading home again.
Whoever you are, no matter how lonely,
the world offers itself to your imagination,
calls to you like the wild geese, harsh and exciting—
over and over announcing your place
in the family of things.

Becoming more aware of what is occurring in moment-to-moment experience may similarly bring a sense of spaciousness. It involves being flexible in attention, noting when attention is focused on one aspect of experience, while maintaining a sense that this narrow focus can be held within a broader field of view. "Staying present" with awareness of the breath, body, sounds, and thoughts is a way to practice taking this wider perspective. We shall see this theme illustrated in different ways as the session progresses: We discuss people's experience, in particular, any feelings of aversion and attachment; we give participants a wider perspective by showing them questionnaires and checklists about the symptoms of depression, and a video of Bill Moyers's documentary of the MBSR program in action (for more information on the video, see Chapter 15); and we introduce them to using the breathing space as a way of handling difficult situations.

HONEYMOONS AND HARD WORK

In reviewing homework week by week, the instructor gets close to the heart of issues that arise with the practice. Even more importantly, the homework review gets close to the heart of the very habits of attachment and aversion that are likely to cause problems. For some people, the "honeymoon" with the program is over and the hard work is beginning.

The following was expressed by someone who had begun to find it hard work because he had become very *attached* to the practice:

"I find I can really get into the practice now. When I'm sitting, I feel in another world. So much so that if anything interrupts, I get really angry. I feel like a child that has had his ice cream snatched out of his hand."

Notice how a pleasant experience has become something to which this person is strongly attached. And the attachment is beginning to produce frustration. Now we are not against pleasant experiences, but it may be worth pausing a moment to explore whether the person was focusing on achieving a "special state" and to be very clear about the intention behind the practice. After exploring the particular situation with the participant, the instructor felt it important to be as clear as possible about this theme:

"It is really nice to hear that you are getting something out of the practice. When we get such pleasant experiences, it can show us that something is happening. But I'm also going to mention here a word of caution. Pleasant experiences may come and go, and while they last, they are wonderful. But the word of caution is this: Sometimes the pleasant experience will not come. Sometimes you may experience unpleasant feelings when you sit. But this won't mean that you are doing badly. It is still meditation, even when it feels bad or boring or frustrating. The task is the same at these times, too: As best you can, be aware of whatever you are feeling right now, and then return your attention to the breath. So although it's really nice when it seems to be going well, if we get hooked on making it always feel like that, our life is going to be a series of ups and downs. We'll have moments of great success, they'll pass, and then what will we do?

"Having this practice gives us a chance to find something that is beyond the ups and downs, beyond the times when things do or don't work out so well for us."

In this case, the instructor invited the participant to look out for similar situations when he felt "attached" to a thought or a feeling, and to note what feelings came up as the situation came and went. Of particular interest is how what is pleasant became a source of frustration (and therefore a negative feeling) the more he tried to cling to what he had judged to be positive.

More often, the hard work comes out of a sense of *aversion* to the homework:

P: I have to come clean and be totally honest. I didn't get round to doing any of the homework. Now I can imagine what R must have felt last week. I felt absolutely terrible myself. You feel as if, you know, you are not even putting the effort in at home, and it's the thin end of the wedge. I feel, you know, I have really let you down.

I: There are two things about that. First taking responsibility for your own homework. There is a relationship between how much homework you do and how you move along—a close relationship. If you don't do it, you reduce the chance of anything happening. This is entirely your responsibility. But second, and the thing I am really interested in, is your feeling of dread and the thoughts about how awful it was going to be coming here. In the course of not doing your homework, all these thoughts come up: about being no good and letting me down, and not coming up to expectations, and so on. Would you like to say some more about that?

P: Well, sitting here right now, with you talking in your calm voice, it's fine, and I'm really glad I came. But then I get a really funny feeling in my stomach and a tightness in my chest because I think you're thinking I'm a failure.

I: This is really important. It's this contrast between the thoughts that you take to be true, and reality. I can give you the reality: I don't feel let down by you. There are no standards. That is not what it's about. It is actually taking the experience as it is, and letting go of all these comparisons. We are moving to the point where you can begin to recognize these thoughts as mental events. "Here come the self-critical thoughts; here come the guilty thoughts; here is the old tape playing again, creating the same feeling." Clearly, these patterns of thinking come from somewhere. It is possible that at some time, you were severely criticized by somebody for not doing things right. But these are old habits. It doesn't matter where they come from. What we are about is trying as best we can to free ourselves of them. The reason why we use the breath focus, with all the long gaps, is simply to give you lots of chances for these thoughts to come in; to give you a chance to say, "Ah, there you are" and gently go back to the breath.

We should not be surprised that aversion and attachment are such common themes in the practice. Each person has his or her own way of handling difficult or painful emotions, whether they arise from memories, current difficulties, or future possibilities. And each person is attached to a huge variety of goals: to have friends, to succeed, to have excitement, to be relaxed. Keeping these basic pluses and minuses in balance is adaptive—they ensure our survival. But much of the time, people find themselves preoccupied with avoiding harm or achieving reward in unhelpful ways that add to the negativity of the unwanted object or event, or to the frustration of not having the object of desire or affection.

These themes often come up again when participants are talking about how they got on with their Unpleasant Events Calendar. Many note that this was easier to complete than the Pleasant Events Calendar. They noticed many more unpleasant moments each day. Once again, we have a blackboard available to write down responses, distinguishing thoughts, sensations, and emotions. We wish to highlight the theme that events may not be inherently positive or negative. It is often the mood state that we bring to events that colors them for us. Second, we wish to note whether people express aversion to the negative thoughts and feelings, taking the opportunity to explore the vicious circles involved in getting upset about having negative thoughts and feelings (e.g., "I should not be feeling like this. Why am I so stupid and weak?").

Note that the theme, which is never very far away from both attachment and aversion, is "wanting things to be different from how they are right now." By contrast, one of the first steps in dealing with our reactions to different mind states is simply to be present with them. This is the most we can ask for at first, and then, in the fuller space of awareness, we may decide how to respond. Learning that we can actually stop struggling and be present gives us the opportunity to see and relate to our circumstances with greater clarity and directness. With this insight comes the possibility of choosing behaviors that are more likely to deal skillfully with the situation before us, rather than having our actions automatically driven by fear or old mental habits.

AUTOMATIC NEGATIVE THOUGHTS AND THE SYMPTOMS OF DEPRESSION: GETTING TO KNOW THE TERRITORY OF THE ILLNESS

One of the most valuable aspects of the structured psychotherapies that developed in the 1960s with behavior therapy and continued with cognitive therapy in the 1970s was the therapists' collaborative approach, their willingness to talk openly and in a matter-of-fact way with patients about how mental health problems can arise and how the aim of therapy is to help them tackle their problems. An important aspect of this was to talk about issues of diagnosis and formulation, about what, in their case, seemed to have caused or maintained the symptoms they were experiencing. Although MBCT does not discuss causes of a particular participant's problems, it retains this important feature: Education about depression is essential if people are going to learn ways to deal with it more skillfully.

At this point, therefore, we move from talking about thinking in general to a more focused discussion of the types of thoughts that are usually reported by people when they are suffering from depression. To help in this work, we used the Automatic Thoughts Questionnaire (see Box 9.4[73]). The questionnaire lists a variety of negative statements (e.g., "I can't get things together," "My life is not going the way I want it to," "What's the matter with me?," "I hate myself"').

The instructor asks if anyone recognizes any of the items from the list. The rationale for the exercise is to provide a sense of the "territory of depression," a view of the disorder as a whole package. The questionnaire includes a space where people can rate both how often they have any particular thought and a space to rate how strongly they believe it. This provides an opportunity for people in the class to reflect on how much their degree of belief has changed since they were depressed. Reading and reflecting on these statements helps people get some distance from these thoughts and to see them as bundled together with a number of other features. This exercise also helps to counter the idea that some of the features of depression are more real than others. For example, some people accept sleep disturbance or problems with appetite and fatigue as signs of a "true depression" but consider feelings of worthlessness, worry, and guilt as signs of a more personal failing. Learning about the full territory of depression helps to integrate parts of the illness that some may consider as separable.

One person's reaction was "I've got them all." Another person immediately started to wonder why her doctor had not recognized her depression earlier. Addressing the instructor, she said: "If you knew that, why don't the GPs? Because this has gone on for years." She thought that if such a questionnaire had been used when she was depressed, then at least it would have shown that someone understood: "If it was in this form, it would prove that someone knows what you felt like. . . . It took me a while to realize that it was depres-

BOX 9.4

⚗️

Automatic Thoughts Questionnaire

Listed below are a variety of thoughts that pop into people's heads. Please read each thought and indicate how frequently, if at all, the thought occurred to you *over the last week*. Please read each item carefully and circle the appropriate answer on the answer sheet in the following fashion (1 = "not at all," 2 = "sometimes," 3 = "moderately often," 4 = "often" and 5 = "all the time"). Then, please indicate how strongly, if at all, you tend to believe that thought when it occurs. On the right hand side of the page, circle the appropriate answers in the following fashion (1 = "not at all," 2 = "somewhat, 3 = "moderately," 4 = "very much," 5 = "totally").

Frequency	Items	Degree of belief
1 2 3 4 5	1. I feel like I'm up against the world.	1 2 3 4 5
1 2 3 4 5	2. I'm no good.	1 2 3 4 5
1 2 3 4 5	3. Why can't I ever succeed?	1 2 3 4 5
1 2 3 4 5	4. No one understands me.	1 2 3 4 5
1 2 3 4 5	5. I've let people down.	1 2 3 4 5
1 2 3 4 5	6. I don't think I can go on.	1 2 3 4 5
1 2 3 4 5	7. I wish I were a better person.	1 2 3 4 5
1 2 3 4 5	8. I'm so weak.	1 2 3 4 5
1 2 3 4 5	9. My life's not going the way I want it to.	1 2 3 4 5
1 2 3 4 5	10. I'm so disappointed in myself.	1 2 3 4 5
1 2 3 4 5	11. Nothing feels good anymore.	1 2 3 4 5
1 2 3 4 5	12. I can't stand this anymore.	1 2 3 4 5
1 2 3 4 5	13. I can't get started.	1 2 3 4 5
1 2 3 4 5	14. What's wrong with me?	1 2 3 4 5
1 2 3 4 5	15. I wish I were somewhere else.	1 2 3 4 5
1 2 3 4 5	16. I can't get things together.	1 2 3 4 5
1 2 3 4 5	17. I hate myself.	1 2 3 4 5
1 2 3 4 5	18. I'm worthless.	1 2 3 4 5
1 2 3 4 5	19. I wish I could just disappear.	1 2 3 4 5
1 2 3 4 5	20. What's the matter with me?	1 2 3 4 5
1 2 3 4 5	21. I'm a loser.	1 2 3 4 5
1 2 3 4 5	22. My life is mess.	1 2 3 4 5
1 2 3 4 5	23. I'm a failure.	1 2 3 4 5
1 2 3 4 5	24. I'll never make it.	1 2 3 4 5
1 2 3 4 5	25. I feel so helpless.	1 2 3 4 5
1 2 3 4 5	26. Something has to change.	1 2 3 4 5
1 2 3 4 5	27. There must be something wrong with me.	1 2 3 4 5
1 2 3 4 5	28. My future is bleak.	1 2 3 4 5
1 2 3 4 5	29. It's just not worth it.	1 2 3 4 5
1 2 3 4 5	30. I can't finish anything.	1 2 3 4 5

Adapted from Hollon and Kendall.[73] Copyright 1980 by Philip C. Kendall and Steven D. Hollon. Adapted by permission.

sion. I just thought I was tired and things were getting me down. . . . .you know, that people like me didn't suffer from depression."

The instructor may suggest that the list can be seen in a number of different ways:

"Here is one way to look at these negative thoughts. Let's see if you can bring some humor to this exercise by picking out a hit list of your favorites. This can be helpful in reminding yourselves that these are just thoughts, not the truth with a capital T. You might also want to take a minute and compare the extent to which these thoughts seemed to be absolutely true when you were feeling depressed, but, at this point, no longer seem to have the same grip.

"Here is another way to look at it. Let's say a common thought you had when you were depressed was 'I'm never going to get over this depression.' Well, we have got the living proof that you did. So these thoughts are absolutely convincing—they just come into your mind—but they are not true. Those are things that drive your feelings; they drive your actions and they are deadly because, if you think you are not going to get over it, if you think you are useless, if you think there is nothing you can do to make any difference, then you give up.

"So we just need to be able to recognize them over and over again and not get sucked into them. The task now is just to learn to recognize them: 'Here are public enemy numbers one to 29' and then you can just say, 'Ah, there you are. I don't need to get sucked into you right now.' "

The second way in which we explore the "territory" of depression, is to study the diagnostic criteria for major depressive disorder from the *Diagnostic and Statistical Manual of Mental Disorders* (DSM-IV-TR; see Box 9.5[26]). These give a clear description of the symptoms that psychiatrists use when diagnosing depression. The reason for going over it is so individuals can recognize that some of the things they may have thought were personal failings are actually bona fide symptoms. Once again, the idea is to give participants another perspective on their symptoms. The message is that depression

---

BOX 9.5

⊗

Diagnostic Criteria for Major Depressive Episode

Has the patient experienced five or more of the following symptoms continuously at least over a 2-week period and in a way that departs from the patient's normal functioning?

1. The patient reports that he or she feels depressed or sad most of the day.
2. There is a loss of interest or ability to derive pleasure from all, or nearly all, activities that were previously enjoyed.
3. Significant weight loss when not dieting or weight gain, or a decrease or increase in appetite nearly everyday.
4. There is difficulty sleeping through the night or the need for more sleep during the day.
5. The patient is noticeably slowed down or agitated throughout the day.
6. The patient reports feeling fatigued or a loss of energy nearly every day.
7. Feelings of worthlessness or extreme, or inappropriate, guilt.
8. The patient reports difficulties with concentration or the ability to think; this can also be seen by others as indecisiveness.
9. Recurrent thoughts of death or ideas about suicide, without a specific suicide plan or a suicide attempt.

Adapted from DSM-IV-TR.[26] Copyright 2000 by the American Psychiatric Association. Adapted by permission.

---

comes as a package of symptoms; the task is to learn how to relate differently to the whole package. Gaining this alternative view of it can go far in preventing people from being trapped in the old, depressive ways of thinking about what it all means.

SOMEWHERE ELSE TO STAND

Note what has happened here. The aim of the fourth session is to explore how to "stay present" in the face of the tendency to chase after the pleasant and avoid the unpleasant. We have seen that this involves giving up old habits in order to allow difficult material to come and go in the mind. But we have introduced the Automatic Thoughts Questionnaire and a symptom checklist of depression. What have these got to do with staying present? The answer is that seeing how the signs and symptoms of depression can change when depression changes, seeing how the negative thinking that comes with it (so strongly believed, so overwhelming when in the depressed state) can change, gives participants "somewhere else to stand" to see more clearly what their minds can do to them. This links with the practice in which participants have been engaged from the outset of the program: to learn to become more aware of body sensations. Learning to "stay present" in the body also presents people with another place to stand. "Staying present" is rarely easy, but it is easier if a person, when his or her mood starts to shift, has a sense that such moods do not last for ever, and that they are part of a recognizable syndrome. The person gains an alternative perspective from which to view his or her experience.

We wanted to give people more opportunity to see things from another perspective, so we built two further elements into this session. First, we made available copies of Jon Kabat-Zinn's book *Full Catastrophe Living* for people to borrow and read between sessions. This book describes the MBSR program. We hoped it would remind people of the things they had done in our classes. It includes the body scan, focusing on the breath, and the yoga. As an accessible guide to the mindfulness approach, it tells in detail stories of people that have gone through MBSR at the UMass Medical Center. But in the context of our program, it reinforces the message that there are alternative perspectives to be had, different ways of seeing what, up until now, many participants have viewed as problems that were unique to themselves.

The other element we build into the session is to play a segment of the Bill Moyers television documentary *Healing from Within* that features the Stress Reduction Clinic at UMass (see Chapter 15). It is helpful because the tape brings to life many of the themes that have already been covered in the program (and that participants will be able to read about in the book). It gives us another chance to review the themes we have explored so far: to see that meditation is about understanding the patterns of the mind; to see more clearly that skillful action follows when we give up wanting things to be different; to see that through watching others learn how to be mindful participants realize that the "chatter of the mind" is both universal and difficult to overcome. Participants may also understand how, in not striving for a perfect solution, it may be possible to learn to see things differently, to get a different perspective on the feelings, thoughts, and body sensations that allows people to live a fulfilling life "around the edges" of the problem that previously overwhelmed them.

We scheduled showing the videotape both in this session and the next. Participants' reports showed that it enabled them to see things from a different perspective. Common comments illustrated themes of solidarity, credibility, the ubiquity of mind wandering, the similarity of tasks for members of both MBCT and MBSR, the need to become more accepting of one's experience, and the importance of nonstriving. Note especially in the following examples how the tape gave participants "another place to stand"—another perspective.

> "I couldn't believe that the other people were saying the same things to themselves about the way their minds were working and how hard it was to get it to stop."

> "Pain is a physical problem, but what we are being asked to do with negative thoughts or sad feelings is really no different."

> "So is the idea that we are not trying to make it all go away, but that, by becoming aware of it, something may change?"

> "The point is not to get somewhere but to be more alive in the present moment."

> "It's almost saying . . . anger is fine, sadness is fine. . . . Let them come and go through the system. It's the clinging to it and going round and round that I need to step away from."

"I am always trying to change how I do things, but some of the people on the tape were happy to leave things alone. They did not try to change or improve how they practiced. They just valued it as it was. I guess the act of just accepting can be an important change in itself."

Both seeing the videotape and the subsequent discussion drew together some important issues that are relevant to the theme of staying present. A central issue is how hard it is to give up striving for things. Persons who practice meditation are not immune to the same strivings. Indeed, it makes it ever more clear. The striving is easily seen when people get rigid about a practice, for example, staying with the breath and not wavering. It does not take much to turn a simple instruction to stay with the breath into a drama of success and failure. It is too easy to believe, deep down, that success is achieved when we are with the breath and failure occurs when the mind wanders. The truth is that meditation is the whole process of staying with the breathing, moving away, seeing that we are no longer on the breath and, then, gently returning. What is important is that we come back without blaming, judging ourselves, or feeling that we have failed. And if we find that we have judged ourselves, then the instruction is still the same: simply to note the judgment and bring attention back to the breath or whatever was the focus of attention.

TAKING A 3-MINUTE BREATHING SPACE DURING CLASS

At the previous session, we introduced the 3-Minute Breathing Space (Handout 8.2) to be used at regular, preset times during the day as a generalization exercise. We now extend the breathing space so it can be used at other times of the day. This involves inviting people deliberately to use the 3-Minute Breathing Space during the week, whenever they notice unpleasant feelings or a sense of "tightening" or "holding" in the body, or of being overwhelmed. At such moments, the breathing space might consist of either taking a full 3

minutes of more "formal" practice or momentarily bringing awareness to what is going on in the mind and body, and with the breath,
during a period of busyness. In the latter case, it is not always possible for participants to close their eyes and make major adjustments to
posture, but the process of intentionally stepping out of automatic pilot remains important. The aim is to use these moments as further opportunities to explore the difference between skillful responding and
automatic reacting.

Given this new use of the breathing space, it is helpful to include
it during the class at appropriate times, in order to bring to bear another mode or perspective. These might be moments when the class
finds itself lost in a lengthy discussion or when strong feelings or reactions surface.

One example of its use is following the videotape, but many
other uses are not so predictable. For example, it is not unusual,
when the class is discussing and analyzing various topics, for everyone's mind (including that of the instructor) to drift away from the
present and off into other thoughts and mental routines. For participants, many of these mental routines simply trigger the old habits of
depressed thinking. During Session 4, in particular, we find that discussing depressive thoughts and symptoms sometimes produces a
sudden sadness in participants. Thinking about depression has the
power to activate a lot of negative thinking. At these times, the
breathing space can help "shift mental gears" and connect with experience in the present moment.

The following is an example of someone who felt sad after he had
read the list of negative thoughts on the Automatic Thoughts Questionnaire:

P: I feel quite sad now, I actually do.

I: About what? Was it reading all this?

P: The thing that got me was . . . because I have spent so much
time. My depressions took a lot of years out of my life. That's
how I feel. . . . It is easy to get back into it. You could easily get
depressed just by looking at this list every day.

I: What we are learning is to how to relate differently to these thoughts and feelings, by practicing over and over again how not to get sucked into them. Why don't we actually do that right now, because there is a sadness in this room, with the thoughts about the previous episodes around. So let's do a breathing space, because it is one of the ways we have to actually come back into the moment. So to start, we could make a quite definite change in our posture . . . sitting upright . . . (*The instructor leads a 3-Minute Breathing Space.*)

This is not done in an avoidant way but rather as a means of acknowledging such feelings, creating space for them, and only then moving to focus on the breath and bring awareness to the body as a whole. The task here is a subtle one. We are not using the 3-Minute Breathing Space to achieve a goal, with the idea that doing this will help a person feel better afterwards. It is really about (1) acknowledging that there is strong feeling around and (2) seeing what happens if we take a moment to bring awareness to it, simply allowing it to be there without judging it, and trying to chase it away or solve the problem. Using it in this way allows people to "touch base," to return to the anchor of the breath wherever they are, to shift mental gears so that they have a different way of investigating how things are for them right at this moment. As a result it may begin to reveal different possibilities, different ways of responding to the variety of mind states. During the week following this class, participants are encouraged to use the 3-Minute Breathing Space not only at set times during the day but also whenever they feel the need for its help in coping with difficulties.

ENDING THE CLASS

The end of Session 4 represents something of a watershed. Given that we are now coming to the halfway point in the course, it is a good idea to review the whole MBCT model with the class before ending with a brief sitting meditation. Given our theme of "staying present," this is an opportunity to emphasize the role of breathing in helping us achieve a different stance toward ourselves, our minds, and our bodies.

People who attend the classes are learning a different way of relating to their entire experience. So when, for example, they are ruminating about letting someone down, or feeling angry with someone, they can use that as an opportunity to practice taking a different, more skillful approach. The transcripts of the MBCT sessions show a similar change taking place:

"For example, I think I started to feel sad because my grandmother is very ill. I kept thinking, 'Oh, I'm getting depressed' . . . but . . . I was saying this to someone just the other day: 'I am sad, I am tired, but I'm not depressed.' And I don't have to deny the sadness or the tiredness."

"Today, I had a difficult phone call to make and, normally, that would go round and round in my mind. I made the phone call, and I was able to deal with the call, but usually, after a conversation like that, I would be worrying about it for ages. But this time, afterwards, it was great. I stopped thinking about it. It didn't carry on and on. Using the breathing space was amazing to me. It seemed to take the worry right away from me, that would have been churning in my mind all afternoon."

These participants are learning to stop and ask the question: "How are things right now?" "What is going through my mind here?" "What is going on in my body?" "What is the most skillful response to make right now?" This inquiring stance itself is becoming for them a reminder to step back and to be a more careful observer of what is going on.

This tiny step can make all the difference. As a result of the practice, people are not simply being drawn in to the "bad feeling"; neither do they have to answer back to their negative thoughts. Instead, they feel able to see themselves and their thoughts and feelings within a wider perspective. They are not separating themselves from their thoughts and feelings entirely, but there seems to be more space in which they can work with them. And with a greater sense of space, they are more able to stay present with whatever they find coming into their minds and be more forgiving with themselves when their best intentions go awry.

⚭

Summary of Session 4: Staying Present

Difficult things are part and parcel of life itself. It is how we handle those things that makes the difference between whether they rule (control) our lives or whether we can relate more lightly to them. Becoming more aware of the thoughts, feelings, and body sensations evoked by events gives us the possibility of freeing ourselves from habitual, automatic ways of reacting, so that we can instead mindfully respond in more skillful ways.

In general, we react to experience in one of three ways:

- with spacing out, or boredom, so that we switch out from the present moment and go off somewhere else "in our heads."
- with wanting to hold on to things—not allowing ourselves to let go of experiences that we are having right now, or wishing we were having experiences that we are not having right now.
- with wanting it to go away, being angry with it—wanting to get rid of experiences that we are having right now, or avoiding future experiences that we do not want.

As we will discuss further in class, each of these ways of reacting can cause problems, particularly the tendency to react to unpleasant feelings with aversion. For now, the main issue is to become more aware of our experience, so that we can respond mindfully rather than react automatically.

Regularly practicing sitting meditation gives us many opportunities to notice when we have drifted away from awareness of the moment, to note with a friendly awareness whatever it was that took our attention away, and to gently and firmly bring our attention back to our focus, reconnecting with moment-by-moment awareness. At other times of the day, deliberately using the breathing space whenever we notice unpleasant feelings, or a sense of "tightening" or "holding" in the body, provides an opportunity to begin to *respond* rather than *react*.

⊗

Homework for Week Following Session 4

1. Practice the Guided Sitting Meditation Tape (Tape 2, Side 1) for 6 out of the next 7 days and record your reactions on the Homework Record Form. (Alternative option: Alternate Guided Sitting Meditation Tape (Tape 2, Side 1) with Yoga Tape (Tape 1, Side 2)—indicate which on the Homework Record Form.

2. 3-Minute Breathing Space—Regular: Practice three times a day, at the times that you have decided in advance. Record each time you do it by circling an R next to the appropriate day on the Homework Record Form; note any comments/difficulties.

3. 3-Minute Breathing Space—Coping: Practice *whenever you notice unpleasant feelings*. Record each time you do it by circling an X for the appropriate day on the Homework Record Form; note any comments/difficulties.

4. Optional: If you have had a chance to view the video *Healing from Within*, you might like to checkout the book of the film—*Full Catastrophe Living*.

HANDOUT 9.3

Homework Record Form—Session 4

Name: ____

Record on the Homework Record Form each time you practice. Also, make a note of anything that comes up in the homework, so that we can talk about it at the next meeting.

Day/date	Practice (Yes/No)	Comments
Wednesday Date:	Tape: R R R X X X X X X X X X X X X	
Thursday Date:	Tape: R R R X X X X X X X X X X X X	
Friday Date:	Tape: R R R X X X X X X X X X X X X	
Saturday Date:	Tape: R R R X X X X X X X X X X X X	
Sunday Date:	Tape: R R R X X X X X X X X X X X X	
Monday Date:	Tape: R R R X X X X X X X X X X X X	
Tuesday Date:	Tape: R R R X X X X X X X X X X X X	
Wednesday Date:	Tape: R R R X X X X X X X X X X X X	

HANDOUT 9.4

Staying Present

Remember to use your body as a way to awareness. It can be as simple as staying mindful of your posture. You are probably sitting as you read this. What are the sensations in your body at this moment? When you finish reading and stand, feel the movements of standing, of walking to the next activity, of how you lie down at the end of the day. Be in your body as you move, as you reach for something, as you turn. It is as simple as that.

Just patiently practice feeling what is there—and the body is always there—until it becomes second nature to know even the small movements you make. If you are reaching for something, you are doing it anyway; there is nothing extra you have to do. Simply notice the reaching. You are moving. Can you train yourself to be there, to feel it?

It is very simple. Practice again and again bringing your attention back to your body. This basic effort, which, paradoxically, is a relaxing back into the moment, gives us the key to expanding our awareness from times of formal meditation to living mindfully in the world. Do not underestimate the power that comes to you from feeling the simple movements of your body throughout the day.

CHAPTER 10

⊗

Allowing/Letting Be

SESSION 5

There is a story told of a king who had three sons. The first was handsome and very popular. When he was 21, his father built a palace in the city for him. The second son was intelligent and also very popular. When he became 21, his father built a palace in the city for him as well. The third son, neither handsome nor intelligent, was unfriendly and unpopular. When he was 21, the king's counselors said: "There is no further room in the city. Have a palace built outside the city for your son. You can have it built so it will be strong. You can send some of your guards to prevent it being attacked by the ruffians who live outside the city walls." So the king built such a palace and sent some of his soldiers to protect it.

A year later, the son sent a message to his father. "I cannot live here. The ruffians are too strong." So the counselors said, "Build another palace, bigger and stronger, and 20 miles away from the city and the ruffians. With more soldiers, it will easily be able to withstand attacks from the nomadic tribes that pass that way." So the king built such a palace, and sent 100 of his soldiers to protect it.

A year later, a message came from the son: "I cannot live here. The tribes are too strong." So the counselors said: "Build a castle, a large castle, 100 miles away. It will be big enough to house 500 soldiers, and strong enough to withstand attacks from the peoples that live over the border." So the king built such a castle, and sent 500 of his soldiers to protect it.

But a year later, the son sent another message to the king. "Father, the attacks of the neighboring peoples are too strong. They have attacked twice, and if they attack a third time, I fear for my life and the life of your soldiers."

And the king said to his counselors, "Let him come home and he can live in the palace with me. For it is better that I learn to love my son than spend all the energy and resources of my kingdom keeping him at a distance."

People who have been depressed in the past have often spent a great deal of effort trying to avoid or push away negative memories, feelings, and experiences. Avoiding unpleasantness and trying to ensure that we minimize discomfort takes (as the king in the story found out) a great deal of effort. Although it can be exhausting, many people feel that the strategy has worked for them in the past, that the energy is worth the exhaustion. Why, then, should they risk adopting alternative strategies?

The theme of this session is to introduce and cultivate the possibility of a radically different relationship to unwanted experience— that of acceptance, allowing, and letting be. The work in the first half of the program has enabled participants to become more aware of where their attention wanders to, to use this awareness to bring them back to the present, and to rely on the breath as the vehicle for moving attention around in these ways. These efforts have allowed a scaffolding to be put into place that will support the work required in the second half of the program, namely, using these skills in the service of preventing relapse and cultivating a different relationship to life more generally. Central to these attempts is the development of a different relationship to experience.

BOX 10.1

⊗

Theme and Curriculum for Session 5

THEME

Relating differently involves bringing to experience a sense of "allowing" it to be, just as it is, without judging it or trying to make it different. Such an attitude of acceptance is a major part of taking care of oneself and seeing more clearly what, if anything, needs to change.

AGENDA

- 40-Minute Sitting Meditation—awareness of breath, body, sounds, thoughts; noting how we relate to our experiences through the reactions we have to whatever thoughts, feelings, or bodily sensations arise; introducing a difficulty within the practice and noting its effects on the body and reactions to it.
- Practice Review.
- Homework Review.
- Breathing Space and review.
- Read Rumi's poem, "The Guest House."
- Watch the second half of the MBSR videotape and discuss.
- 3-Minute Breathing Space—Coping and review.
- Distribute Session 5 participant handouts.
- Homework assignment:
  Sitting meditation 6 out of 7 days (use tape days 1, 3, and 5; use no tape days 2, 4, and 6, sit with silence).
  3-Minute Breathing Space—Regular (3 times a day).
  3-Minute Breathing Space—Coping (whenever you notice unpleasant feelings).

PREPARATION AND PLANNING

- In addition to your personal preparation remember to bring the *Healing from Within* video and the poem "The Guest House" to class.

(cont.)

PARTICIPANT HANDOUTS

Handout 10.1. Summary of Session 5: Allowing/Letting Be.
Handout 10.2. Using the Breathing Space—Extended Instructions.
Handout 10.3. Homework for Week Following Session 5.
Handout 10.4. Homework Record Form—Session 5.

CULTIVATING A DIFFERENT RELATIONSHIP TO EXPERIENCE

A relationship to experience that is characterized by acceptance/allowing/letting be is not easy to describe or to cultivate. In preparing ourselves for this task, it is helpful to keep three questions in mind: What is the flavor of acceptance/allowing/letting be? Why is it important in preventing relapse? How can it best be cultivated or used?

WHAT IS THE FLAVOR OF ACCEPTANCE?

At first sight, many participants find "acceptance" a very difficult idea to grasp. Is not acceptance the same thing as resignation? In fact, it turns out that the opposite is true. Acceptance means actively responding to feelings by *allowing* or *letting be* before rushing in and trying to fix or change them (the more common response). Allowing these feelings to be in awareness means that participants register their presence before deciding how to respond to them. This takes a conscious commitment and the deliberate deployment of energy. Resignation, on the other hand, implies passivity and a degree of helplessness. Such difficulty in getting across the flavor of acceptance illustrates the limitations of single words as vehicles to convey the essence of a particular stance or relationship to experience.

Poetry can be used as an alternative vehicle for communicating this different relationship to experience. For example, consider the attitude of active acceptance that is expressed simply and profoundly in the poem "The Guest House" by Rumi, a 13-century Sufi poet.

BOX 10.2

⊗

"The Guest House"

This being human is a guest house.
Every morning a new arrival.

A joy, a depression, a meanness,
some momentary awareness comes
as an unexpected visitor.

Welcome and entertain them all!
Even if they're a crowd of sorrows,
who violently sweep your house
empty of its furniture,

still, treat each guest honorably.
He may be clearing you out
for some new delight.

The dark thought, the shame, the malice.
meet them at the door laughing,
and invite them in.

Be grateful for whoever comes,
because each has been sent
as a guide from beyond.

From Barks and Moyne.[77] Copyright 1995 by Coleman Barks and John Moyne. Originally published by Threshold Books. Reprinted by permission of Threshold Books.

We read "The Guest House" in full during Session 5 to illustrate just how radical a shift we seek. Here is someone speaking about assuming a positive relationship to unwanted feelings with phrases and words such as "welcome," "treat each guest honorably," "invite them in," "be grateful." Is this attitude even possible? Might we actually cultivate a basic friendliness to *all* experiences, including the most difficult and feared?

Even if we find such a stance difficult to imagine, making even a tentative first step in this direction can be invaluable and transformative. This involves meeting things, including our strong emotions, as they are, letting go of any attempts to show them the door.

Embarking on the next step, to take a stance of meeting each and every thought, feeling, or bodily sensation "at the door laughing" is even more radical. It goes against our tendency to distinguish between and react differently to the things we enjoy on the one hand, and those we dread on the other. Saki Santorelli[76] echoes this when he writes that "the poem may be suggesting an inner attitude toward whatever we encounter, urging us to consider the possibility of meeting our grief and pain open handedly. This is not our usual way of meeting adversity" (p. 151). Most of the time, the effort we put into our impulse to resist, avoid, or withdraw keeps us from seeing that an alternative approach is possible. This striking presentation of an alternative approach is one of the things that is so valuable about this poem.

WHY IS THE CULTIVATION OF ACCEPTANCE/ ALLOWING/LETTING BE IMPORTANT?

Acceptance is so important because its opposite is too risky. An unwillingness to accept negative feelings, physical sensations, or thoughts (due to aversion) is the first link in the mental chain that can rapidly lead to the reinstatement of old, automatic, habitual, relapse-related patterns of mind. We see this every time someone says "I'm stupid to think like this" or "I should be strong enough to cope with that." By contrast, to bring *intentionally* an alternative relationship of acceptance/allowing/letting be to unwanted experiences has effects on a number of fronts. First, by encouraging us to pay attention more intentionally, it serves to offset the tendency for our attention to be automatically "hijacked" by passing thoughts or moods. Second, it shifts the basic stance toward experience, from one of "not wanting" to one of "opening." This allows the chain of conditioned, habitual responses, to be broken at the first link. Third, it gives the person a chance to see whether his or her thoughts are accurate, are telling the truth. Consider a thought such as "If this goes on any longer, I'm going to scream." Allowing it simply to be there and, as best we can, noticing the effects it has on the body and seeing the moment-by-moment changes in its intensity may offer us the chance to see that the thought may fade. Its dire prediction did not come true. We shall have more to say about how to deal with thoughts in Session 6.

HOW CAN WE CULTIVATE AND USE ACCEPTANCE/ALLOWING/LETTING BE?

Much of the previous discussion illustrates the difficulty of purely cognitive or effortful attempts to change our basic stance or relationship to experience. Patients frequently may have been admonished to be more loving, caring, and accepting, but the question remains, how to do it? These qualities are unlikely to be produced merely by an effort of will. In this session, therefore, we examine an alternative route for learning to relate differently: working through the body by bringing our attention/awareness to manifestations of difficult experience.

As part of the sitting meditation practice at the start of this session, we introduce explicit instructions that contrast the practice of the previous sessions with that of the current session. We point out that

> "Up to now, the practice has been one of using the breath or body as the focus of attention. The intentional task has been to bring awareness to the sensations of the breath as it moves in and out of the body. Inevitably, our awareness and attention stray from the breath to other thoughts, bodily sensations, and feelings. When this occurs, the instructions up to now have been simply to notice where the mind is, then gently and firmly escort awareness back to the breath, and continue to maintain awareness focused on the movement of the breath."

But what do we do when our awareness repeatedly gets pulled in the same direction, to a particular thought stream, feeling, or set of bodily sensations? What is being asked of us when the pull on our attention is strong and our minds keep going back to the same place?

One way to begin "opening to the difficult" is to think of the practice as having two steps. The basic approach remains to become mindfully aware of whatever is most predominant in one's moment-by-moment experience. So, if the mind is repeatedly drawn to a particular place, to particular thoughts, feelings, or bodily sensations, then the instructions are, to bring awareness deliberately and intentionally to that place. That is the first step.

The second step is to bring awareness to how we are relating, *in the body*, to whatever arises in that place. At this point in the practice, we introduce the idea of acceptance, starting with its opposite, nonacceptance:

> "We can 'be with' an arising thought, feeling, or bodily sensation, but in a nonaccepting, reactive way. If we like it, we tend to hold onto it; to want it to stay; we become attached to it. If we do not like it because it is painful, unpleasant, or uncomfortable in some way, we tend to contract, to push it away out of fear, irritation, or annoyance; we want it to go. Each of these responses is the opposite of acceptance.
>
> "One way to relate skillfully to unpleasant experiences is to register that they are here, to allow them to be as they are, in this moment, and simply to hold them in awareness. Responding in this way, described as 'allowing,' 'letting be,' or 'holding in awareness,' conveys the core theme of acceptance toward difficult feeling states. This is in contrast to automatically reacting to these thoughts or emotions."

DELIBERATELY BRINGING THE DIFFICULT/ PROBLEMATIC TO MIND

At this point, whenever possible we use problems that arise naturally in the course of the program as opportunities to practice this different way of relating to inner experience. These problems can be excellent "grist for the mill" and this is why we welcome expressions of boredom and irritation from participants earlier in the program. Embodying such a welcoming attitude can itself feed a general shift in one's relationship to the difficult. But if no such experiences arise, then what we ask in this session is that participants intentionally bring a problem to the "workbench of the mind" in order to practice relating differently to it. Again, doing this intentionally creates the implicit message: The purpose is not to get rid of your difficulties.

The meditation practice begins by orienting participants to acceptance/allowing/letting be:

> ". . . the easiest way to relax is to stop trying to make things different. Accepting experience means simply allowing space for whatever is going on, rather than trying to create some other state. Through acceptance, we settle back into natural awareness of what is present. We let it be—we simply notice and observe whatever is already present. This is a new way to deal with experiences that have a strong pull on our attention."

We then instruct participants to bring to mind difficult issues, with the aim of noting where in the body they are felt:

> ". . . so now, focusing on some troubling thought or situation— some worry or intense feeling; noticing the feelings that arise in your body.
> ". . . becoming mindfully aware of those physical sensations . . . deliberately moving your focus of awareness to the part of the body where those sensations are strongest. Using the breath as a vehicle to do this—just as you practiced in the body scan, directing your awareness to that part of the body—'breathing into' that part of the body on the inbreath."

Having identified where in the body the physical sensations are the strongest, we can become aware of any aversion present by investigating where in the body the manifestations of such an attitude are expressed. It is then possible to begin observing the physical sense of resisting, holding, pushing away, or tensing and bracing. These body sensations are first brought into awareness, and then a sense of "opening" and "softening" on the outbreath is brought to them, in order to work on the second step, *letting go of aversion*:

"Once your attention has moved to the bodily sensations and you have the item in the field of awareness, saying to yourself, 'It's OK. Whatever it is, it's OK. Let me feel it.' Then just staying with the awareness of these bodily sensations and your relationship to them, breathing with them, accepting them, letting them be. It may be helpful to repeat 'It's OK. Whatever it is, it's OK. Let me feel it.' Softening and opening to the sensations you become aware of. Saying to yourself, 'Soften,' 'Open,' on each outbreath."

The instructions allow participants to stay with this aspect if they wish:

"Keeping your awareness with those bodily sensations and your relationship to them so long as they have a pull to attract your attention. Perhaps holding together in awareness both the sensations and the sense of the breath—breathing with the sensations. When you sense that the bodily sensations are no longer pulling for your attention, simply returning 100% to the breath and continuing with that as the primary object of attention."

Finally, we include instructions for doing this aspect of the practice if participants notice no reaction in the body to the difficult experience:

"If, in the next few minutes, no powerful bodily sensations arise, try this exercise with any bodily sensations that you notice, even if they have no particular charge."

In this way, the practice aims to explore the consequences of reversing the habitual tendency of the mind to move *away* from the painful/difficult. This is done through intentionally bringing awareness (a gentle, kindly, friendly awareness) *to* the sense of how the difficult is manifesting *in the body*, including aversion-related physical sensations. In this way, one can begin to reverse one's habitual rejection of the difficult and the unpleasant, and cultivate an attitude of acceptance and friendliness. Bringing a gentle curiosity to something is, itself, part of acceptance. Holding something in awareness is an implicit affirmation that we can face it, name it, and work with it. Also, letting go of aversion in the body may be easier and more relevant to the needs of participants who have been depressed, because it provides an alternative to an approach based on thoughts. Focusing on the body may help participants avoid getting caught up in ruminative patterns of thinking.

We find it helpful to support this inner work with detailed suggestions for exploring edges, watching the intensity go up and down, *breathing into* as ways to carry awareness, supported by words such as "it's OK" and invitations to feel it. These all add up to a package of friendship rather than hostility toward experience. The stance of the instructor is obviously crucial if this is to take place with any authenticity.

BUT IT IS DIFFICULT

Consider the difficulty that one person reported when we talked about this aspect of the practice in the class:

P: I find it difficult to say "It's OK" over some things. Because when you say "it's OK," it's not OK. It has to do with noise from the dogs that belong to the people next door. The dogs aren't actually theirs. They belong to their parents-in-law, but they look after them when their in-laws go away. It happened again today. They were barking and barking. They keep them tied up outside when they go out, and even sometimes when they are in, and they bark and howl all day long.

I tried the breathing and, in the end, I just had to leave the house. It was no use. I kept ringing them up and getting the answer machine. I hammered on the door. Nobody answered. I just had to go out in the end. Now, I find it very difficult with something as invasive as that to say, "it's OK." I couldn't deal with it today at all.

I: The words are simply meant to be a way to help you in that particular moment to come to a point of balance. It is not actually the final decision on the state of the world. There's a story in a book written by a famous American teacher of meditation. He was in India, and after a great deal of effort, he found himself the ideal little house perched up in the mountains, and he booked it for a few months of absolute peace and stillness for a retreat. The day after he had got himself settled in there, a couple of hundred yards down the hill, a group of Girl Guides arrived and set up loudspeakers on poles all the way round and played pop music full blast from 6 A.M. to 10 P.M.

P: I bet they had dogs, too!

I: Dogs and pop music; and all through loudspeakers! He suffered the same experience as you. It took days and weeks before he could say, "That's just the way things are just now." Acceptance is not something you can immediately turn on. It's really making some gesture toward not immediately triggering a range of automatic responses.

Clearly, this participant was not only having a difficult time with her neighbors, but also she could not see how coming to the classes was going to help. Note, however, that it was not just the noise that was upsetting, but her own reaction to it. In some ways, the classes were in danger of contributing to the sense that she was not handling it very well:

P: I felt I failed because I hadn't coped with it. I did the breathing, and I did everything else; and then I just had to go out, because I couldn't get on with anything. And I thought: "This is a failure, running away from it"; but it was the only thing I could do at that moment.

We can see here that, in addition to the problem of the noise, she had noticed her reaction and judged herself harshly for it. She was "failing" by running away from it. The instructor picked up on this point.

I: This is very very important. It may really have been the only thing you could do, but was it a failure? This is the thing to hone in on. The reason for telling you about the man in India was that he couldn't immediately cope with it either. That is just how it is sometimes, so adding "This is a failure" is extra and can create more problems for you.

P: Yes. What was getting to me was that there were several things that I needed to do and to get on with in the house. Every time I called and got the answering machine, a sort of rage came over me.

I: You may not be able to do anything about the noise, I mean, once you have done everything you can, phoned them, knocked on the door, and nothing has happened; but you still have the possibility of doing something about your internal state.

P: I agree. This is why I am still here, to be honest; because I found that doing this breathing exercise meant that the turmoil didn't go on for so long, you know. This is what I found. When I came back, and it was quiet, I wasn't on tenterhooks all the time, thinking "God, when is it going to start again." That's a good point.

I: You know, acceptance, which is the name of the game we are talking about here, is very difficult to cultivate. But it is something that we may benefit from tremendously if we simply remember to cultivate it as best we can in any moment.

WORKING THROUGH THE BODY

It is natural to be concerned that the instruction to bring to mind deliberately a difficult situation might do more harm than good. But our reasoning is that just as yoga practice gives people the opportunity to work with bodily sensations that have been induced by the stretches, so our participants may need experience at working with negative thoughts and moods (and their consequences in the body) that they have deliberately brought to mind. Feedback from participants suggests that they find this very helpful. Consider how, in a report from a class of our colleague, Surbala Morgan, one participant was able (after some struggle) to bring a difficult thing to mind, then to work with it in the body (by bringing awareness to it, breathing into it, and discovering a wider space within which it could exist). We pick up the session where the participant was discussing her reaction to the request to bring to mind a difficult thought.

P: When you said it, I thought, "I'm not sure I'm going to be able to do this. I can't think of anything." And I got worried that I was going to miss out on this exercise. Then, suddenly, something came up into my mind. It was to do with our son, who has been giving us a really hard time recently—staying out all hours, hanging around with people we don't trust. We had a real crisis 2 months ago involving the police. As soon as this came into my mind, I knew it was going to be difficult to get out of my mind again. I try not to think about it at all, but every time I do, I think, "Where have I gone wrong?"

The next instruction, to become aware of what was happening in the body, took her even more deeply into a place she did not want to be.

P: And then, when you said, "How do you feel physically?", that was quite dreadful. And I realized that that is exactly how I feel when I think about what's happening in the family. And then you said, "What is your body doing?" At that moment, it was as though my breathing stopped completely. And you were saying, "Recognize what's tense." And I thought, "Yes, it's all tense around here."

Then, a change occurs. The instruction is given to bring awareness to and to breathe into the place in the body that is most tense. This was something of a transformative experience for her.

P: And then when you said to breathe into it, that was really good, because it was giving it space. Before, it was like the whole of my body around here was really tight and knotted. And then you said. "Breathe into it," and it suddenly became like a great big empty space . . . with the air coming in and out. You know, sometimes when you come back from holiday, and the house is a bit musty, so you open all the doors and windows to let the air blow through . . . well, it was like that . . . having doors and windows open, and with curtains blowing and air coming in and out. And it was really amazing. And the tension about my son was still there, you know. I thought, "Oh, you're still there, but never mind, the wind's blowing through and that's alright."

I: So although it was still there, there was more space?

P: Mmm. Yes, and I could sort of look at it. The feeling in my body was still a bit tight, but it was much smaller, and all the air was sort of flowing around it. At the beginning, it was the whole thing. Because I was so tight, you know, there was nothing else there.

The instructor was then able to use this participant's experience to illustrate one of the central themes of the mindfulness approach, and the participant responded by giving a graphic description of the reduced size of the problem, and indicated an increased willingness in the future to explore an alternative to pushing difficult things away.

I: This is exactly what we're about here. This is a really good example. Because it's not about trying to get rid of these states. There's always going to be something going on. There's always going to be something distressing or difficult. And it's not about not having the feelings that go along with those difficult states, but it's exactly as you described—having more space around the feelings, so that there's the discomfort, the distress, and there's more of you, and there's breathing there as well.

P: To begin with, it was like a solid mass of rock. It was huge. It was so solid that you couldn't get around it, but then it shrank to a small stone. It was still stone . . . but it was small. It's really good. Because I think, probably, I have been pushing the issue away and sort of sitting on it, and not letting it come up fully to the surface. I haven't allowed it before to simply be there. I thought it would just overwhelm me.

I: It felt as if it would take you over or . . . ?

P: Yes, I think so. Yes, it probably would take me over. It was too much to let in and so my natural reaction, well, before this course, would have been just to tense and push it away, and not even to face it.

I: And now . . .

P: And now—now I've got all this air under there.

I: This is lovely, isn't it? So in a sense, it's less scary that these things are there. It's still not pleasant, you know. It would be nice if you could get rid of all the negatives. But it's not possible. But you're now more able to allow them to be here and not feel crushed by them.

P: Yes, and I started thinking, "Oh, I might like to do that again, just to try it again," which is quite amazing because in the past I would never think, "Ah, I'll have that feeling again."

I: Mmmm. It's very different then. Remember the poem about welcoming each guest across the threshold? It's like you're becoming more welcoming to all different sorts of states.

P: Yes.

IS THIS "ACCEPTANCE," OR A CLEVER WAY TO FIX THINGS?

One of the most subtle and difficult issues is how to bring an accepting attitude to something without having the hidden agenda of "fixing" it. The distinction between fixing and accepting is a difficult one to grasp, perhaps because when people talk about accepting something, they often describe positive changes that they have noticed as a result. Acceptance is then linked to positive outcomes, so it is natural then to try to reproduce such a positive outcome and use "acceptance" as part of "doing/driven" mode, as a means of achieving the goal of relaxation or happiness. In the following transcript, we read that Katie, a professional fund-raiser, sees herself as making progress in dealing with some work-related stress. At first it seems that an old style of coping, by distraction and pushing away, seems to have made things easier for her. Rereading the transcript with the theme of this session in mind, however, it is clear that, at some level, she used the focus on the breath to fix a difficult situation, without any real shift toward a relationship of acceptance.

> "There was this person at work doing some rather silly things. I work for a fund-raising business. He was drafting a job description for a new post, but he hadn't given it to the personnel department to look at. I was trying to explain the procedure he must go through; otherwise, we don't have the authority to advertise the post. He could not see this. I was getting more and more worked up, and I thought to myself, "No, I've got to try and just concentrate and get my mind off it and concentrate on my breath.' And I did that, and my mind went back on it again, and I said, 'No, come on back,' and it went back. And it was like a shuttle service! But I did notice this, which rather pleased me. Instead of it going on for an hour winding up, it didn't. This is what I was quite pleased with. It took a while (don't get me wrong), but then I thought to myself, "No, I'm not thinking about that anymore. It's not continually going on.' "

The danger is that using the breath to escape, fix, or avoid things tends not to make for a lasting change. Consider the following comment:

> "Concentrating on the breath again, it took me away from the bad feelings, and then I started thinking, 'Oh, I've got a lot of things that really cause my depression,' and I moved to all of them very quickly and I started feeling a bit 'ugh.' "

At other times, however, it was clear that the practice was changing some more fundamental aspect of how a person related to difficult experiences. In going to visit his father following a routine surgical procedure, Michael reported:

> "I was going to visit my father in the hospital last Monday. You never know what you are going to find when you get there . . .

you get so many mixed messages. So early Sunday morning, I woke up feeling really apprehensive and panicky. So I thought, 'Unpleasant event, unpleasant event, unpleasant event,' right, which I haven't actually done before. I thought, 'Breathe in to relax.'"

Note that, up to this point, Michael appears to be using the breath to relax, to fix his stress. Then a change occurs:

". . . but in fact, I thought, 'Now, what are you really feeling?'" I was really pleased because I was thinking, 'My tummy's churning, my hands are clenched. I'm having difficulty with breathing.'"

By making use of the "acknowledging" step of the breathing space, bringing awareness intentionally to body sensations, Michael was able to bring a more gentle, friendly attitude to what was going on.

". . . and then I started breathing . . . and it didn't progress on . . . it didn't progress on. I was really pleased because what it does is make you feel that everything isn't out of control. After all, it doesn't solve everything straightway—those things were still there—but it did help. It did help."

BREATHING SPACES

We can see by these comments that some people begin to explore the 3-Minute breathing space as a way to pause and gather themselves in the midst of troubling situations. It begins to allow some people the chance of seeing a problem (and what might best be done about it) more clearly, rather than getting caught up in older, more depressive ways of viewing things. Our intention for the breathing space is that, if possible, it should always be more than taking a time-out. By encouraging people to step out of automatic pilot, to become aware of the "here and now" of their breath and body sensations, there can be a change in the quality of the awareness of feelings or thoughts: a freshness of perspective that allows people to take a wider view of their experience rather than getting caught up in it.

Once again, the idea is to focus on awareness of body sensations that accompany any intense thought or emotion. This makes it more likely that, should a thought or feeling seem overwhelming, the person would be able to bring awareness to what is most difficult *as it is felt in the body*. From now on, however, participants are encouraged to add a sense of "opening to the difficult" within the breathing space. In addition to the basic instructions for Step 3, the following, further instructions might now added:

> "Allow your attention to expand to the whole body—especially to any sense of discomfort, tension, or resistance. If these sensations are there, then, bring your awareness there by 'breathing in to them' on the inbreath. Then, breathe out from those sensations, softening and opening with the outbreath. Say to yourself on the outbreath, 'It's OK to feel this way,' 'It's OK, whatever it is, it's OK. Let me feel it.' "

A Note of Caution

Participants vary in the ways in which they use the coping breathing space. Some people see it as an "escape hatch," a brief moment when they can retreat and relax before advancing again into the busyness of their lives. Others see it as an opportunity to bring awareness to what is going on at that moment, to notice and step out of the routine they have become caught up in, so that they might relate differently to the difficulty awaiting them. There is some evidence that the first strategy, though it gives short-term benefits, is not helpful in the long run, perhaps because it does not alter the person's perspective on what gives rise to the feeling of stress and pressure. The second strategy proves to be a more skillful approach to using the breathing space. What is going on here?

An example might help. Most of us have at some time been caught in a severe downpour of rain and have run for shelter, perhaps in a telephone booth or shop doorway. Sometimes we have simply been glad to be out of the rain. We stand for a while, hoping it will stop. We are dry at the moment, but as the rain continues, we know that sooner or later we are going to have to face it; the thing we tried to escape is still there. We may go back out into the rain, cursing it gently as it drenches us. At other times, we may take shelter in a different way. We stand for a while, aware of being wet and not liking it much. We notice that we are hoping it will stop, but see that it shows no sign of stopping and realize that we are going to get wet. We note that being upset about it only adds to our discomfort. We stop clinging to the hope that it will stop raining. Doing this allows us to look more closely at the rain itself. There is something rather compelling about the way it is splashing off everything it hits. We go back out into the rain. It has not stopped, but our relationship to it has changed the whole experience.

Does this mean that if we take the first approach, and find ourselves cursing the rain, we have "failed the test"? Not at all, because nobody is immune to such feelings. They are just the next opportunity to see how best to relate to experience. Just as we can welcome difficult things at the door of the guest house, we can also put out the red carpet for feelings of failure—even failure to welcome the last guest! This is a shameless red carpet! Learning to relate differently in this way takes a great deal of practice, however. The effort it takes is illustrated in the second half of the video, *Healing from Within*.

MINDFULNESS AND CHRONIC PAIN

The second half of the MBSR videotape describes the approach that patients in the program learn for working with problems such as chronic pain, hypertension, or anxiety. We are introduced to a patient with chronic back pain due to three separate accidents that each damaged his spine. Why show a video featuring someone with chronic pain to a class of people who have come to learn how to prevent depression? It turns out that the themes of "allowing" and "letting be" are critical in both. Participants in MBCT find no difficulty in seeing the connection. This provides the instructor with further opportunities to underline certain key messages.

"... the main change was not that the pain was actually eliminated, but that the distress from the pain was reduced: The key
phrase in all this is relating differently to what you've got. It's
saying, 'OK, you're here. Let me come in close. Open the guest
house; roll out the red carpet.' "

This very concrete example gives us a great opportunity to examine the issue of how best to relate to difficult things:

"There are some situations, like chronic pain, where acceptance
may be the most skillful thing you can do. There are other situations (depression is clearly one of them) where there are things
you can do. Nonetheless, the first step is always acceptance, relating differently to it, because that first step is often enough to
see what action will be most helpful to take."

Even more interesting are the possible links between the theme
of relating to the difficult and the persistent idea that all these techniques (even those that say they are not) are simply more subtle ways
of fixing things. This theme came up earlier in the session, but it is so
important it bears repeating.

"Last week, when we were talking about breathing into the difficult, I was trying to fix it. That's what I was trying to do. In one
way, it's physical, but the mental part, if you like, is 'OK, it's a
pain; OK, that's what going on.' If you extend that into things
like depression and anxiety, and take a kindly interest, then it's a
fine line between acknowledging that's what it is and not making
it worse by fighting it, and finding a way of breathing into it, but
without the intention of getting rid of it."

In reading this transcript, it is clear that here is someone who is
getting right to the heart of one of the most radical challenges that
MBCT presents.

"You've put your finger on it. I mean, that is absolutely what it's
about, and it's difficult. The most natural tendency in the world

is to pretend: "I won't tell that I'm doing this; I'll just take a kindly interest in it; I'm not really going to fix it.' But . . . we end up trying to fix it anyway."

She had hit on one of the main themes underpinning the entire program: that inasmuch as we tend to try to fix our problems (however subtly), we run the risk getting caught in the loop in which we match ourselves against some ideal standard, then find ourselves (and our attempts to fix things) falling short. If this occurs, it puts us back in the "doing/driven" mode and we are likely simply to end up ruminating about how, if meditation doesn't "work," perhaps we have reached the end of the road and had better give up everything. MBCT is based on the radical (in the sense of going to the root) notion that the best way "to get somewhere" is not to try and get anywhere at all, but to open to the way things actually are in this moment; that direct perception and observation will show us new ways of navigating outside the "box" of our habitual patterns of reacting, seeing, and thinking about things.

ENDNOTE

The story of the king and his three sons, with which we began this chapter, did not say how things ended. The king had realized that keeping his son at a distance used up too many of his resources. That was the first step. But we are left wondering whether he was simply resigned to having to tolerate his son, or whether he had made a fundamental shift toward "welcoming" the difficult, altering radically his relationship with those things in his life that caused him pain and hardship. The ambiguous ending invites the question: Which of these possible attitudes was more likely to bring the king lasting peace?

Summary of Session 5: Allowing/Letting Be

The basic guideline in this practice is to become mindfully aware of whatever is most predominant in our moment-by-moment experience. So if the mind is being repeatedly drawn to a particular place, to particular thoughts, feelings, or bodily sensations, we deliberately and intentionally take a gentle and friendly awareness to that place. That is the first step.

The second step is to notice, as best we can, how we are relating to whatever arises in that place. Often, we can be with an arising thought, feeling, or bodily sensation, but in a nonaccepting, reactive way. If we like it, we tend to hold onto it; we become attached. If we do not like it, because it is painful, unpleasant, or uncomfortable in some way, we tend to contract, to push away out of fear, irritation, or annoyance. Each of these responses is the opposite of acceptance.

The easiest way to relax is, first, to stop trying to make things different. Accepting experience means simply allowing space for whatever is going on, rather than trying to create some other state. Through acceptance, we settle back into awareness of what is present. We let it be—we simply notice and observe whatever is already present. This is the way to relate to experiences that have a strong pull on our attention.

For example, if you notice that your awareness keeps being pulled away from the breath (or other focus of attention) to particular sensations in the body associated with physical discomfort, emotions, or feelings, the first step is to become mindfully aware of those physical sensations, to deliberately move your focus of awareness to the part of the body where those sensations are strongest. The breath provides a useful vehicle to do this—just as you practiced in the body scan you can take a gentle and friendly awareness to that part of the body by "breathing into" that part on the inbreath, and "breathing out" from it on the outbreath.

Once your attention has moved to the bodily sensations and you have the item in the field of awareness, say to yourself, "It's OK. Whatever it is, it's OK. Let me feel it." Then, just stay with the awareness of these bodily sensations and your relationship to them, breathing with them, accepting them, letting them be. It may be helpful to repeat, "It's OK. Whatever it is, it's OK. Let me feel it," using each outbreath to soften and open to the sensations of which you become aware.

Acceptance is *not* resignation: Acceptance, as a vital first step, allows us to become fully aware of difficulties, and then, if appropriate, to *respond* in a skillful way rather than to *react* in knee-jerk fashion, by automatically running off some of our old (often unhelpful) strategies for dealing with difficulties.

Using the Breathing Space—Extended Instructions

When you are troubled in thoughts or feelings:

1. AWARENESS

Observe—bring the focus of awareness to your inner experience and notice what is happening in your thoughts, feelings, and bodily sensations.

Describe, acknowledge, identify—put experiences into words, for example, say in your mind, "A feeling of anger is arising" or "Self-critical thoughts are here."

2. REDIRECTING ATTENTION

Gently *Redirect* your full attention to the breath.

Follow the breath all the way in and all the way out.

Try noting "at the back of your mind," "Breathing in ... breathing out" or counting, "Inhaling, one ... exhaling, one; inhaling, two ... etc."

3. EXPANDING ATTENTION

Allow your attention to expand to the whole body—especially to any sense of discomfort, tension, or resistance. If these sensations are there, then take your awareness there by "breathing into them" on the inbreath. Then, breathe out from those sensations, softening and opening with the outbreath. Say to yourself on the outbreath, "It's OK. Whatever it is, it's OK. Let me feel it."

Become aware of and adjust your posture and facial expression.

As best you can, bring this expanded awareness to the next moments of your day.

Homework for Week Following Session 5

1. Practice Sitting Meditation daily (alternate days: Tape 2, Side 1; no tape—sit with silence for 30–40 minutes) and record your reactions on the Homework Record Form.

2. 3-Minute Breathing Space—Regular: Practice three times a day at times that you have decided in advance. Record each time by circling an R next to the appropriate day on the Homework Record Form; note any comments/difficulties.

3. 3-Minute Breathing Space—Coping: Practice *whenever you notice unpleasant feelings*. Record each time by circling an X for the appropriate day on the Homework Record Form; note any comments/difficulties.

※

Homework Record Form—Session 5

Name: _____

Record on the Homework Record Form each time you practice. Also, make a note of anything that comes up in the homework, so that we can talk about it at the next meeting.

Day/date	Practice (Yes/No)	Comments
Wednesday Date:	Tape: R R R × × × × × × × × × × ×	
Thursday Date:	Tape: R R R × × × × × × × × × × ×	
Friday Date:	Tape: R R R × × × × × × × × × × ×	
Saturday Date:	Tape: R R R × × × × × × × × × × ×	
Sunday Date:	Tape: R R R × × × × × × × × × × ×	
Monday Date:	Tape: R R R × × × × × × × × × × ×	
Tuesday Date:	Tape: R R R × × × × × × × × × × ×	
Wednesday Date:	Tape: R R R × × × × × × × × × × ×	

CHAPTER 11

⚹

Thoughts Are Not Facts

SESSION 6

John was on his way to school.
He was worried about the math lesson.
He was not sure he could control the class again today.
It was not part of a janitor's duty.

What do you notice as you read these sentences? Most people find that, as they move from one to the next, they have to "update" the scene in their mind's eye. First of all, it is a little boy going to school, worried about the math lesson. Suddenly, the scene changes. For most people, the "mental model" changes to a teacher, before it finally changes into the janitor. It illustrates clearly the fact that we make an implicit inference around the bare facts we are reading. We are actively "making meaning" out of the sensory input all the time, and we are barely conscious that we are doing so, until someone comes along and plays a trick on us, as in this series of sentences. It is almost as if the mind creates a running commentary on all the events that take place in our awareness.

It is easy to see how these inferences, these "commentaries" that occur in our minds, may create or maintain emotional reactions. Once we have made the inference, the emotion follows close behind it. A phone call from a friend might be interpreted as "She needs me" or as "She's using me," and our reaction will be completely different depending on which it is. Or imagine the following domestic scene: A husband and wife are in the kitchen. "Would you like fish or soup for supper?," says one. "I don't mind," says the other. Now we shall leave to one side the inference we have all already made about who is asking the question and who is giving the answer! But imagine that they go for counseling because they have some marital difficulties. She remembers that event as "I asked him whether he would like fish or soup for supper, and he said he didn't care." He remembers that event as "She asked me what I wanted, and I said that I would like anything that she cooked for me; I was trying to be helpful." Note again how easily the same event can have different interpretations.

This problem in separating events from interpretation of events can cause a big problem for many people. People who are vulnerable to depression often interpret events in ways that are self-denigrating. Their thoughts become like propaganda directed against themselves. Facts are mixed with self-deprecating thoughts in a very destructive way, resulting in conclusions such as "I am worthless" or "I am a failure" or "If people knew what I was really like, no one would want to know me." And once such an internal propaganda stream has started, it is very difficult to undermine it, for all future events will tend to reinforce it: Contrary information is ignored; consistent information is noticed.

DEALING WITH THOUGHTS IN COGNITIVE THERAPY AND MINDFULNESS-BASED COGNITIVE THERAPY

Until the advent of cognitive therapy for depression in the 1970s, the role of such self-directed, negative propaganda in causing and maintaining depression had been ignored by many therapists. The fact that depressed people had such negative thoughts was obvious, but clinicians assumed that they were caused *by* the depression—the result of underlying biological, psychodynamic, or behavioral processes. Cognitive therapists thought differently: Unremitting nega-

BOX 11.1

⊗

Theme and Curriculum for Session 6

THEME

Negative moods, and the thoughts that accompany them, restrict our ability to relate differently to experience. It is liberating to realize that our thoughts are merely thoughts, even the ones that say they are not.

AGENDA

- 40-minute sitting meditation—awareness of breath, body, sounds, then thoughts (plus noting reactions to introduction of difficulties).
- Practice Review.
- Homework Review (including sitting meditation without tape and breathing spaces).
- Mention preparation for end of course.
- Moods, thoughts, and alternative viewpoints exercise.
- Breathing space and review.
- Discuss breathing space as the "first step" before taking a wider view of thoughts.
- Distribute Session 6 participant handouts and Series 2 tapes.
- Homework assignment:
  Practice with selection from Series 2 tapes for a minimum of 40 minutes a day.
  3-Minute Breathing Space—Regular (three times a day).
  3-Minute Breathing Space—Coping (whenever you notice unpleasant feelings)

PREPARATION AND PLANNING

- In addition to your personal preparation remember to bring materials for the alternative viewpoints exercise and the Series 2 tapes to class.

(cont.)

PARTICIPANT HANDOUTS

Handout 11.1. Summary of Session 6: Thoughts Are Not Facts.
Handout 11.2. Ways You Can See Your Thoughts Differently.
Handout 11.3. Homework for Week Following Session 6.
Handout 11.4. Homework Record Form—Session 6.
Handout 11.5. When You Become Aware of Negative Thoughts.
Handout 11.6. Relating to Thoughts—I.
Handout 11.7. Relating to Thoughts—II.

tive thoughts could cause depression. Interpreting events in the most pessimistic and hopeless way had a number of psychological consequences: It reduced self-esteem, increased guilt, interrupted concentration, and undermined social interaction. In addition, such thinking could have biological consequences (poor appetite, disrupted sleep patterns, agitation or retardation). Once in place, these symptoms themselves would provide even more evidence for the negative self-propaganda, more evidence of the person's stupidity, weakness, or worthlessness.

Cognitive therapy revolutionized the treatment of depression. Its core feature was working to help patients take their thoughts and interpretations seriously, to "catch" their thoughts and write them down, then gather evidence for and against them with an open mind. These procedures, applied systematically with homework exercises to give extended practice at the skills, were found to reduce depression in ways that would have been astounding to clinicians in the 1950s and 1960s.

In both its rationale and its practice, cognitive therapy puts an explicit emphasis on the content of thoughts. For example, a depressed women who believes 100% that "my friends are sick of me" will be encouraged by the therapist to think of this as an idea (an hypothesis) that may be true or false but needs to be tested against the evidence of recent events and future homework experiments. Eventually, she may be able to "answer back" the negative thought. In this case, she may be able to say "I haven't seen my friends because both I and they have been really busy, not because they are sick of me" or "I had meant to see Nicky last weekend, but I was out of town."

A critical test of whether the reality testing has worked is the degree of belief in the thought before and after the evidence has been examined. But our analysis of how cognitive therapy has its lasting effects (see earlier chapters) suggested that this patient would be less likely to relapse if, during the course of her therapy, she changed the relationship to her thoughts; that is, although the *explicit* emphasis had been on changing the content of her thoughts through challenging them, answering them back, seeking evidence for and against their truth value, we suggested that changes needed to take place at another level, a level that was left *implicit*. The patient needed to begin to shift her relationship to thoughts, to recognize her thoughts as thoughts.

SITTING WITH THOUGHTS AS THOUGHTS

What is implicit in cognitive therapy is made explicit in MBCT: this need for a change in relationship to one's thoughts and the entire process of thinking. A key objective of Session 6 is to help participants find ways of reducing their degree of identification with what they are thinking, to encourage them to see thoughts as thoughts (even the ones that say they are not). Our aim is to enable participants to shift their relationship, so that they no longer relate *from* their thoughts but *to* their thoughts, as objects of awareness.

By this point in the MBCT program, this message has been conveyed implicitly hundreds of times. Participants have had a lot of practice noticing their mind wandering, labeling what is going on in their minds as "thinking." They have, many times, gently brought the focus of attention back to the breath, or body, or whatever the intended focus. Sometimes the thoughts were trivial, sometimes not so trivial. Many thoughts, noticed during practice at home, were temporarily compelling, simply because they seemed to demand immediate action: "I ought to phone Mary before I forget," "Was that someone at the door?," "Will I remember to give Bob that report tomorrow?" The less trivial ones seemed compelling because they "meshed" with a prevailing negative mood and seemed to be absolutely true as a result: "I can't do this. I may as well give up," "When he said that, I know he meant something more by it," "There's so much to do at work, I'll never get it all done." In each case, the instruction was the same: to note where the mind had gone and gently bring it back to the breath. The message was implicit: This is just a thought. In this way, participants were learning to step back, to decenter from the content and just notice the thoughts.

Now we wish to make the relationship with thought more explicit: to make thoughts the objects of awareness. In the sitting meditation that starts the session, we take the opportunity to pay particular attention to observing and recognizing thoughts as thoughts, to bring awareness to them as discrete mental events, and to see each thought as simply a thought, an idea in the mind. We use the phrase "thoughts are not facts" to suggest that we don't have to believe everything we think or take it as absolute truth.

> "Taking a few moments now to become aware of the thoughts that are arising in your mind, imagine yourself sitting in a cinema. You are watching an empty screen, just waiting for thoughts to come. When they come, can you see what exactly they are and what happens to them? Some of them will vanish as you become aware of them."

Note the "waiting" for thoughts to come. The attitude of mind is rather like that of a cat, patiently and attentively waiting at the mouse hole for any sign of movement. But much of the time, our attention is anything but cat-like.

Joseph Goldstein[74] offers a helpful analogy:

> When we lose ourselves in thought, thought sweeps up our mind and carries it away, and in a very short time we can be carried far indeed. We hop a train of association not knowing that we have hopped on, and certainly not knowing the destination. Somewhere down the line we may wake up and realize that we have been thinking, that we have been taken for a ride. And when we step down from the train, it may be in a very different state of mind from where we jumped aboard. (pp. 59–60)

As in Session 5, as part of the practice in this session, we encourage participants to bring to mind deliberately some concern, difficulty, or unpleasant memory—to become aware of and briefly bring to mind any thoughts that go along with it. In this exercise, participants practice bringing awareness, a gentle interest, to their thoughts as they arise in the field of awareness. Some participants find the metaphor of the cinema screen very helpful, but others find different metaphors and analogies useful. Some see "thoughts" come onto an empty stage and exit through the opposite wing. Others find it helpful to think of their mind as the sky, with clouds moving across it at varying speeds. Sometimes the clouds might be small; at other times, they are dark and looming, covering the entire sky. But the sky remains. Toward the end of this session, we distribute more mindfulness meditation practice tapes (Series 2 of Jon Kabat-Zinn's tapes; see Chapter 15), which include both mountain and lake meditations. These guided meditations offer helpful images that convey vivid ways of relating to thoughts, such as the mountain that stays grounded even though stormy weather rattles around it, or the lake bottom that stays calm even though the water's surface is disturbed by wind and rain.

STANDING BEHIND THE WATERFALL

So far, the emphasis has been on bringing awareness to one's thoughts. But sometimes, the thoughts are so negative that to bring awareness to them directly seems too difficult. If this happens, we have a number of options. First, we might bring our awareness to a place where such thinking might be having an impact on the body.

"If there is a place in the body that is experiencing intense sensation, then bringing your awareness to that region. Surrounding the physical sensations with a sense of friendly interest.

"Perhaps, on each outbreath, saying, 'It's OK. Whatever it is, it's OK.' Soften and open to the sensations you are experiencing. Particularly if there's any sense of resistance, bringing gentle awareness to it, on each outbreath, opening and softening as best you can, rather than tensing or bracing.

"When it feels comfortable, returning the focus to the breath or to the body as a whole."

Second, since many thoughts are closely tied to particular feelings, we might focus directly on the feeling that gives rise to the thought. For example, if the thought is "I'm so useless at everything; I never finish anything," we risk being dragged down by a powerful waterfall of ruminations about the consequences of failure. However, instead of getting tangled in thoughts, we have the option of asking, "What is this I am feeling now, specifically, in this moment?" In this case, we may discover more feelings than were apparent earlier: *"I am feeling very anxious, worried, tense, angry and frustrated, uncertain and confused as well."* Focusing on the feelings that partly drive the vicious cycle of thoughts may give us another place to stand. We may find ourselves standing behind the cascading waterfall of negative thoughts and feelings, and able to see their force more clearly without being dragged down by them.

An example of the way this might sometimes help came in the experience of Louise, the participant we mentioned in Session 2 (Chapter 7). She had some difficult weeks when she felt very low: she knew that, normally, she would spiral downward again. On one such occasion, she was in the doctor's surgery with one of the children. She felt pressured because she had had to take time off work to be there, thinking not only "What will the boss say?" but also "Why shouldn't I be here? I'm entitled to it," and so on and on.

She noticed what was happening, but not in the old way, when she dealt with it by telling herself not to be so stupid. Instead, she took a moment. She acknowledged what she was feeling: angry, tired, confused, and very worried about her child. Then she felt her perspective broaden and found herself able to say, "It's OK to feel like this; it's OK." She allowed the feelings just to be there, without struggling to chase them away. They dissipated in a way that she later called "miraculous." She had never before experienced anything like that in her life.

So both cognitive therapy and MBCT emphasize that thoughts

are best seen as events in the mind, events to which we are ordinarily so close that it is often difficult to realize they are "just thoughts." Mindfulness gives this different relationship to thoughts a more explicit focus. It does not emphasize gathering evidence for or against them, nor answering them back, as a first step in gaining distance from them. Instead, it encourages people to bring a different mind, a different quality of attention to bear upon them; to observe them as part of a whole package that, although we do not know where it has come from, now needs to be acknowledged and treated with an attitude of gentleness and acceptance. In this way, we can reduce some of the effort that we have expended in dealing with them, as if they were telling the truth about the world or ourselves, the past, or the future. We also stop allowing ourselves to be controlled by them or, at least, we begin to see the tendency for that to happen emerge in the present moment. Once we see negative thoughts from this perspective, from behind the cascading waterfall, our emotional response to them will be different in subtle but important ways.

SEEING THE "TAPE IN THE MIND" FOR WHAT IT IS

The meditation teacher Larry Rosenberg[71] points out that when we get to the point where we've watched the mind a great deal and seen the same old thoughts come up again and again, we don't rise to the bait anymore: "It's like seeing *Gone with the Wind* for the fifth time or the twelfth, however many it takes you. The first eleven were great, but the twelfth doesn't work anymore. You just don't care. The same thing happens with the movie in your mind, if you really start to watch it" (p. 142).

Naming our favorite thought patterns is one way that helps us to recognize them when they are starting up. It allows us to say, *"Ah, I know this tape, this is my 'I can't stand my boss' tape or 'No one recognizes how hard I work' tape."* This will not necessarily switch it off, or if it appears to, it will almost certainly return soon, like a children's movie at holiday season. The difference will be in the way we relate to it: as "fact" that should be addressed seriously on the one hand; for example, by phoning the boss and complaining to him or her, or on the other hand, as a tape running in the head that will continue to be a minor inconvenience until the "batteries run down" and it ceases of its own accord.

Such a stance toward our own thoughts does not come naturally, and for people who have been depressed, certain thoughts can be so powerful that seeing them as simply thoughts can be a huge challenge in itself. Furthermore, many people do not experience their minds as having "thoughts" as such. They may "think" in images or pictures. For example, if they feel rejected by their friends, they may not have the thought "My friends are sick of me." They may simply see, in their mind's eye, a picture of their friends huddled in a corner, laughing and talking among themselves.

Many participants notice that bodily sensations often seem to be magnets for thoughts. Thoughts may arise as a reaction to an awareness of sensations: "Why am I feeling this way?", "It's my age. I'll never have the energy I used to have," "If this headache doesn't go away, I will have to cancel my plans for tonight." To approach these thoughts mindfully does not require that we do anything different than what we have been doing up to now for sensations and feelings. We can imagine we are in a cinema or theater and simply decide to watch the film or theater of the mind as thoughts come and go on the screen or stage. However, we also point out that this is not easy to do, and it should be practiced for only 3 or 4 minutes at a time in the early stages.

When we practice mindfulness at home, we cannot avoid noticing a range of negative thoughts and images that are often very self-critical and reactive. In the week preceding this session, participants were invited to try formal practice without using a tape on certain days. This proved difficult for some, who found that they simply could not concentrate. Notice how this difficulty was compounded by thoughts: First, that previous weeks were so good that now participants were disappointed, and second, that if they could not do it "well," it was useless to do it at all:

P: I had a dreadful week, a really dreadful week. I didn't do any meditation and I didn't get round to reading any of the book. The weeks before were so good, I was really getting into it. I just can't concentrate on anything at all at the moment.

I: What do you think was going on?

P: I really don't know. I think it is just loneliness. I have been busy, but I was making time before. I was consciously making time because I enjoyed it. It was my time.

I: Right, but when you needed it most, you lost it?

P: Yes. There were a couple of times in the week when I tried to do it at work, and I just couldn't do it. My mind wouldn't concentrate. It was constantly running.

In this case, a *fact* (that her mind was constantly running) was mixed with an *interpretation* (this means "I couldn't do it"). There is a choice here for the instructor. He could have pointed out the fact/interpretation issue or addressed what the practice actually demands. He decided to do the latter first.

I: That's OK. I think what is really important, particularly at times like this, is not to assume that you have got to sit down and be able to "do it properly." Simply sitting down for the allotted time and watching your mind race is much better than not doing it at all, even though it is not so easy to bring yourself to practice in such circumstances. But these are some of the best times to practice. The truth is, if you look back with the benefit of hindsight, you can see that the times you just sat with all that stuff raining down on you have actually been as or more valuable than the times when you have been peaceful and calm.

Later, the instructor found the opportunity to rediscuss the way that thoughts get mixed up with facts.

I: Often when we are practicing and the mind is all over the place, we find ourselves getting angry and frustrated. The thoughts and feelings seem like a huge waterfall, and we feel as if we are being hurled down with the force of the water. At these times, as best you can, see if you are able to stand behind the waterfall. Watch the thoughts and feelings, including the understandable frustration you feel. The thoughts and feelings cascade past you. They are very close. You can feel the force of them but they are not you.

All of these points may arise out of discussion of both the sitting meditation practice at the start of the session and the homework. Recall that participants have practiced using the 3-Minute Breathing Space regularly during the day and taking a breathing space whenever difficult things come up. This will become an increasingly important "scaffold" for dealing with difficulties, including negative thoughts, and we return to it later. For now, we wish to explore another way of illustrating the core theme of this session: the alternative ways to relate to thoughts.

WHEN MOODS AND THOUGHTS CONSPIRE AGAINST SEEING ALTERNATIVE VIEWPOINTS

Our colleague Isabel Hargreaves devised the following moods and thoughts exercise, which demonstrates to participants some of the ways in which feelings can determine how we think about a particular situation (it is adapted here by permission of Isabel Hargreaves). The instructor gives each person a piece of paper with a scenario written on it: version 1 on the front of the paper, and version 2 on the back. Participants write down what they would think, first using version 1, then version 2.

Version 1 says: "You are feeling down because you've just had a quarrel with a colleague at work. Shortly afterward, you see another colleague in the General Office and he or she rushes off quickly, saying he or she couldn't stop. What would you think?"

Version 2 says: "You are feeling happy because you and a work colleague have just been praised for good work. Shortly afterward, you see another colleague in the General Office and he or she rushes off quickly, saying he or she couldn't stop. What would you think?"

In the discussion that follows, class members compare the thoughts and feelings brought up by each description. It's not un-

usual to hear that the first situation is associated with thoughts of being rejected or hurt by the colleague's hurrying away, while in the
second scenario, the colleague's rushing off may draw out thoughts of
curiosity or concern for his or her welfare, or the thought that he or
she might be jealous. For example:

P: In the first case, it would keep going over in my mind, why my
       colleague hadn't spoken to me, whereas in the other one, I would
       just accept it without another thought.

I: So we have got exactly the same objective situation [the actual
       evidence is that the person said he or she couldn't stop and
       rushed off], but at least to some of us, the frame of mind we bring
       to it creates a radically different interpretation, a different set of
       feelings. This makes the very obvious point that just because we
       think something doesn't make it so.
           Thoughts carry credibility. We believe them. But we have
       this capacity to make all these different interpretations of the
       same situation, so that if these are going to be determined by the
       frame of mind that we bring to it, and we are in a negative frame
       of mind, we are in danger of getting trapped in the interpreta-
       tions that frame of mind produces, and our mood gets worse, and
       then down we go.
           So the first stage is really to get thoroughly aware of this dif-
       ference between thoughts and facts. Part of the point of medita-
       tion is to perceive this distinction; we note our thoughts as pass-
       ing events in the field of awareness; we note their content and
       their "emotional charge," and then we bring our attention back
       to the breath. As best we can, we do not get caught in the
       thought stream. We just say, "Oh, there's another thought; then,
       we go gently but firmly back to the breath."

The important point here is that interpretation of events reflects
what we bring to it as much or more than what is actually there. We
have already seen how what we think can influence how we feel, but
the new element here is that what we think is also determined by our
mood at the time we are thinking. The idea that *thoughts are not facts*

is as relevant to people who have recovered from depression as to those who are still depressed. Discussing how the same event can be interpreted differently, depending on what happened immediately beforehand, suggests that there is no single truth that our thoughts are telling us. This exercise suggests that thoughts are interpretations that reflect a number of different influences, including learning from our past and current mood states. Just because our thoughts are compelling does not make them true.

SO WHAT IS THE FIRST STEP?

Participants need to feel that there is something they can do immediately, when they feel their thoughts getting the better of them. We therefore emphasize that taking a breathing space (no matter how briefly) is always the first step. Bringing awareness to the breath, a person has a greater chance of acknowledging what is going on with him- or herself at this moment. With this awareness often comes the sense of a greater choice about how to respond. One picture we have in mind is that the breathing space is like a door. Opening the door reveals a number of different corridors down which we might decide to go.

The critical thing is to become aware that there is a choice. In the next session, we consider how people can choose to take action following a breathing space. Here, we focus on how best to deal with thoughts. But the message remains: Take a breathing space as a first step.

Once that has been done, there are a number of options as to what to do next. First, participants might use some of the tools developed by cognitive therapists for people who become aware of trains of thoughts that have a strong emotional charge.[78] These are included in the participant handouts for people to try on their own:

1. To simply watch your thoughts come and go in the field of awareness, without feeling that you have to follow them.
2. To view all your thoughts, and particularly negative thoughts, as mental events rather than facts. It may be true that a par-

ticular thought "event" is often associated with strong feelings. It is therefore tempting to think of it as being true. But it
is still up to you to decide to what degree it is true, if at all,
and how you want to deal with it.

3. To write your thoughts down on paper. This lets you see them
   in a way that is less emotional and overwhelming. Also, the
   pause between having the thought and writing it down can
   give you a moment to reflect on its meaning.
4. To ask yourself the following questions: "Did this thought just
   pop into my head automatically?", "Does it fit with the facts
   of the situation?", "Is there something about it that I can
   question?"

With time, participants may begin to see thinking as an activity
on its own, and just note when it is happening. This reveals the process of thinking as it unfolds, but without participants' getting lost in
its content or what the thoughts are trying to say. If participants can
relate to their experience of thinking in this way, it may enable them
to choose between those thoughts they wish to act on and those they
can simply let be.

A fundamental point is that if we are able to recognize our self-
talk in this way, we place ourselves in a better position to *choose* what
we want to do about it. If, when we notice an avalanche of thinking,
we take a breathing space, there are a number of things we can do
next, if need be. These include not only observing our self-talk, or
writing it down, but also bringing our awareness to the feelings behind it, as best we can, with an attitude of gentleness: "There may be
other ways to see this."

Finally, paying such careful attention to our sensations and
thoughts can give us a moment to take a different view of our difficulties, so that they become less stressful. For example, if we are criticized by our boss at work, instead of letting it snowball into insecu-
rity or defensiveness, with mindfulness, we can watch our initial
reactions go by before we speak, then speak more consciously and
therefore more effectively.

The important point is that *all thoughts are mental events (including the thoughts that say they are not!).*

A "DIFFERENT RELATIONSHIP TO THOUGHTS" IS NOT JUST ANSWERING THEM BACK

Many people report that using the breathing space as a first step in dealing with negative thinking proves very helpful. But we must be cautious. There is a subtle but important difference between using the breathing space to try and strengthen us to fight against the thoughts versus standing in a different relationship to them. In the first case, simply trying to find more and more clever answers to negative thoughts may leave us with a greater sense of hopelessness.

Note, in the transcript that follows, how this person moves from simply trying to "answer back" her negative thoughts in the first part, to simply seeing them as thoughts in the second. In particular, notice the dangers of using the "answering back" mode; it too easily lapses back into self-criticism, while the "seeing thoughts as thoughts" mode brings a different tone.

P: I know from the start when I'm having a bad day.

I: It starts the moment you wake up?

P: Yeah, well, I can have a good start and it can deteriorate throughout the day, but sometimes, first thing in the morning, it's one of those days. Sometimes I get increasingly frustrated with myself for not being able to do what I think I should be able to do. That's when reminding myself that it's not my fault and it will be better in the next day or in the next couple of hours is helpful.

I: So you challenge some of your thoughts with those thoughts?

P: Yeah, and I use the breathing space for that sort of thing . . . and for things that have happened in the past that are of no consequence, or shouldn't be of any consequence. Things somebody said that weren't meant to hurt suddenly hurt, you know. They had no intentions to hurt and I shouldn't take them to heart, you know. I'll suddenly think of something that somebody said 2 weeks ago. "I bet she meant such and such," "Why did she say that?" and my mind just races and races.

I: It can pick up on small things?

P: Really and, you know, it's stupid. There is no sense whatsoever in having that thought and keeping it going round and round in your head. It just does it.

Notice that, at this point, it looks as though this person is using the breathing space as a sort of tool to "pull herself together." The struggle to keep on terms with her negative thinking is very evident, and a tendency to use self-criticism is clear from comments such as "It's stupid" and "There's no sense whatever in having that thought." But later, it becomes clearer that the Breathing Space does connect her to other aspects of the classes:

P: I also think of that saying—"Thoughts aren't facts," was it? That one really clicked with me. "Thoughts are not facts" and the other bit that said ". . . even the ones that tell you they are." I thought that was really good (*laughs*)—"Thoughts are not facts even the ones that tell you they are"—because if you've got that sort of thing going around in your head, you can say, "Now come on. That is not real. This is real. You're here in this room and look at all the good things that are around you." And then the other thought would come back in. "But she really did say that. That really did happen." And then I was able to pick up on the next phrase, ". . . even the ones that say they are" (*laughs*). Then I do the breathing space and I usually find that it's gone.

PREPARING FOR THE FUTURE

At the end of this session, there are only two classes left. At this point, therefore, we allow time for participants to explore their own way of making the practice part of their daily lives. To help them, we make available a collection of mindfulness meditation practice tapes (the Series 2 tapes of Jon Kabat-Zinn; see Chapter 15). The Series 2 tapes include 10-minute, 20-minute, and 30-minute sitting and lying down practices, as well as two guided visualization meditations (involving imagery of a lake and a mountain), and a tape with only the sound of bells at intervals to provide minimal structure for a person's own practice. Given the theme of this session, participants might find either the mountain or lake meditations particularly helpful, since they explore the theme of "being with" negative thoughts and feelings, without completely identifying with them. But participants are asked to choose their own selection from the Series 2 tapes and practice a minimum of 40 minutes per day. This might involve using the 20-minute tapes twice a day or a 30-minute and 10-minute tape over the course of the day.

The implicit message here is that by offering the opportunity to explore these different means, we invite participants to settle into long-term practice. Mindfulness is a way of life rather than a short-term therapy that will "cure" whatever has "gone wrong" with the person. The more people can incorporate formal practice into their lives, and make it as routine as brushing their teeth or taking a bath or shower, the more likely the change that has begun during the 8-week program will continue. It is the "everydayness" of the practice that is important, not exactly which practice is used or for how long. Some people will hear the message "Unless I continue for 40 minutes a day, I will not stay well." This is not what we wished to imply. But we are more and more convinced that it is important to be clear about the future: Putting time aside on a daily basis to sample the "being" rather than "doing" mode is one of the most helpful gifts that people can give to themselves.

※
Summary of Session 6:
Thoughts Are Not Facts

Our thoughts can have very powerful effects on how we feel and what we do. Often those thoughts are triggered and run off quite automatically. By becoming aware, over and over again, of the thoughts and images passing through the mind and letting go of them as we return our attention to the breath and the moment, it is possible to get some distance and perspective on them. This can allow us to see that there may be other ways to think about situations, freeing us from the tyranny of the old thought patterns that automatically "pop into mind." Most importantly, we may eventually come to realize deep "in our bones" that *all thoughts are only mental events* (including the thoughts that say they are not), that *thoughts are not facts*, and that *we are not our thoughts*.

Thoughts and images can often provide us with an indication of what is going on deeper in the mind; we can "get hold of them," so that we can look them over from a number of different perspectives, and by becoming very familiar with our own "top ten" habitual, automatic, unhelpful thinking patterns, we can more easily become aware of (and change) the processes that may lead us into downward mood spirals.

It is particularly important to become aware of thoughts that may block or undermine practice, such as "There's no point in doing this" or "It's not going to work, so why bother?" Such pessimistic, hopeless thought patterns are one of the most characteristic features of depressed mood states, and one of the main factors that stop us taking actions that would help us get out of those states. It follows that it is particularly important to recognize such thoughts as "negative thinking" and not automatically give up on efforts to apply skillful means to change the way we feel.

∞

Ways You Can See Your Thoughts Differently

Here are some of the things you can do with your thoughts:

1. Just watch them come in and leave, without feeling that you have to follow them.

2. View your thought as a mental event rather than a fact. It may be true that this event often occurs with other feelings. It is tempting to think of it as being true. But it is still up to you to decide whether it is true and how you want to deal with it.

3. Write your thoughts down on paper. This lets you see them in a way that is less emotional and overwhelming. Also, the pause between having the thought and writing it down can give you a moment to reflect on its meaning.

4. Ask yourself the following questions: Did this thought just pop into my head automatically? Does it fit with the facts of the situation? Is there something about it that I can question? How would I have thought about it at another time, in another mood? Are there alternatives?

5. For particularly difficult thoughts, it may be helpful to take another look at them intentionally, in a balanced, open state of mind, as part of your sitting practice: Let your "wise mind" give its perspective.

Based in part on Fennell.[78]

⊗⊗

Homework for Week Following Session 6

1. Practice with your own selection from the Series 2 tapes a minimum of 40 minutes a day (e.g., 20 + 20, 30 + 10, etc.). Record your reactions on the Homework Record Form.

2. 3-Minute Breathing Space—Regular: Practice three times a day at times you have determined in advance. Record each time by circling an R on the Homework Record Form; note any comments/difficulties.

3. 3-Minute Breathing Space—Coping: *Whenever you notice unpleasant thoughts or feelings* (paying particular attention to *thoughts*)—If negative thoughts are still around after the breathing space, then write them down. You might like to use some of the ideas in Handouts 11.2 and 11.5 to get a different perspective on these thoughts. Record each time you use the 3-Minute Breathing Space—Coping by circling an X for the appropriate day on the Homework Record Form; note any comments/difficulties.

4. Note situations in which you use the breath as an anchor to *handle the situation as it is happening,* and situations in which you use the mindfulness practice to *deal with the issues later.*

Homework Record Form—Session 6

Name: _____

Record on the Homework Record Form each time you practice. Also, make a note of anything that comes up in the homework, so that we can talk about it at the next meeting.

Day/date	Practice (Yes/No)	Comments
Wednesday Date:	Tape: R R R × × × × × × × × × × ×	
Thursday Date:	Tape: R R R × × × × × × × × × × ×	
Friday Date:	Tape: R R R × × × × × × × × × × ×	
Saturday Date:	Tape: R R R × × × × × × × × × × ×	
Sunday Date:	Tape: R R R × × × × × × × × × × ×	
Monday Date:	Tape: R R R × × × × × × × × × × ×	
Tuesday Date:	Tape: R R R × × × × × × × × × × ×	
Wednesday Date:	Tape: R R R × × × × × × × × × × ×	

When You Become Aware of Negative Thoughts

When you become aware of negative thoughts and images in your mind, hold them in awareness, with an attitude of gentle interest and curiosity, perhaps expanding awareness to include one or more of the following (go back to the breath after each one):

Perhaps I am confusing a thought with a fact?

Perhaps I am jumping to conclusions?

Perhaps I am thinking in black-and-white terms?

Perhaps I am condemning myself totally because of one thing?

Perhaps I am concentrating on my weaknesses and forgetting my strengths?

Perhaps I am blaming myself for something that isn't my fault?

Perhaps I am judging myself?

Perhaps I am setting unrealistically high standards for myself, so that I will fail?

Perhaps I am mind reading/crystal ball gazing?

Perhaps I am expecting perfection?

Perhaps I am overestimating disaster?

The keynote attitude to take with your thoughts is gentle interest and curiosity.

Relating to Thoughts—I

It is remarkable how liberating it feels to be able to see that your thoughts are just thoughts and not "you" or "reality." For instance, if you have the thought that you must get a certain number of things done today and you don't recognize it as a thought, but act as if it's "the truth," then you have created in that moment a reality in which you really believe that those things must all be done today.

One patient, Peter, who'd had a heart attack and wanted to prevent another one, came to a dramatic realization of this one night, when he found himself washing his car at 10 o'clock at night with the floodlights on in the driveway. It struck him that he didn't have to be doing this. It was just the inevitable result of a whole day spent trying to fit everything in that he thought needed doing today. As he saw what he was doing to himself, he also saw that he had been unable to question the truth of his original conviction that everything had to get done today, because he was already so completely caught up in believing it.

If you find yourself behaving in similar ways, it is likely that you will also feel driven, tense, and anxious without even knowing why, just as Peter did. So if the thought of how much you have to get done today comes up while you are meditating, you will have to be very attentive to it as a thought or you may be up and doing things before you know it, without any awareness that you decided to stop sitting simply because a thought came through your mind.

On the other hand, when such a thought comes up, if you are able to step back from it and see it clearly, then you will be able to prioritize things and make sensible decisions about what really does need doing. You will know when to call it quits during the day. So the simple act of recognizing your thoughts as thoughts can free you from the distorted reality they often create and allow for more clear-sightedness and a greater sense of manageability in your life.

This liberation from the tyranny of the thinking mind comes directly out of the meditation practice itself. When we spend some time each day in a state of nondoing, observing the flow of the breath and the activity of our mind and body, without getting caught up in that activity, we are cultivating calmness and mindfulness hand in hand. As the mind develops stability and is less caught up in the content of thinking, we strengthen the mind's ability to concentrate and to be calm. And if each time we recognize a thought as a thought when it arises and register its content and discern the strength of its hold on us and the accuracy of its content, then each time we let go of it and come back to our breathing and a sense of our body, we are strengthening mindfulness. We come to know ourselves better and become more accepting of ourselves, not as we would like to be, but as we actually are.

⊗

Relating to Thoughts—II

The thinking level of mind pervades our lives; consciously or unconsciously, we all spend much or most of our lives there. But meditation is a different process that does not involve discursive thought or reflection. Because meditation is not thought, through the continuous process of silent observation, new kinds of understanding emerge.

We do not need to fight with thoughts or struggle against them or judge them. Rather, we can simply choose not to follow the thoughts once we are aware that they have arisen.

When we lose ourselves in thought, identification is strong. Thought sweeps our mind and carries it away, and, in a very short time, we can be carried far indeed. We hop a train of association, not knowing that we have hopped on, and certainly not knowing the destination. Somewhere down the line, we may wake up and realize that we have been thinking, that we have been taken for a ride. And when we step down from the train, it may be in a very different mental environment from where we jumped aboard.

Take a few moments right now to look directly at the thoughts arising in your mind. As an exercise, you might close your eyes and imagine yourself sitting in a cinema watching an empty screen. Simply wait for thoughts to arise. Because you are not doing anything except waiting for thoughts to appear, you may become aware of them very quickly. What exactly are they? What happens to them? Thoughts are like magic displays that seem real when we are lost in them but then vanish upon inspection.

But what about the strong thoughts that affect us? We are watching, watching, watching, and then, all of a sudden—whoosh!—We are gone, lost in a thought. What is that about? What are the mind states or the particular kinds of thoughts that catch us again and again, so that we forget that they are just empty phenomena passing on?

It is amazing to observe how much power we give unknowingly to uninvited thoughts: "Do this, say that, remember, plan, obsess, judge." They have the potential to drive us quite crazy, and they often do!

The kinds of thoughts we have, and their impact on our lives, depend on our understanding of things. If we are in the clear, powerful space of just seeing thoughts arise and pass, then it does not really matter what kind of thinking appears in the mind; we can see our thoughts as the passing show that they are.

From thoughts come actions. From actions come all sorts of consequences. In which thoughts will we invest? Our great task is to see them clearly, so that we can choose which ones to act on and which simply to let be.

Adapted from Goldstein.[74] Copyright 1993 by Joseph Goldstein. Adapted by arrangement with Shambhala Publications, Inc., Boston, www.shambhala.com.

CHAPTER 12

❦

How Can I Best Take Care of Myself?

SESSION 7

Anna worked as a secretary during the day but took an avid interest in ice skating and attended many classes at night. She especially enjoyed going to competitions with her classmates and had one coming up on the weekend. Anna was also under a lot of stress at work and had been telling herself that she was capable of doing a better job. As she dressed for a skating session, she became aware of thinking that she was not a very good skater and had little chance of scoring well in the competition.

In the past these thoughts would have overwhelmed her. Many times over the past few years, she had given up enjoyable activities because she thought that taking time for herself was self-indulgent. Especially when there was pressure at work, Anna felt that she ought to spend all her available time doing extra tasks for the firm.

This time, Anna became aware of her low mood and decided to take a breathing space. She described becoming aware of and acknowledging what was on her mind, then bringing her attention to her breathing. Finally, she expanded her attention to the body as a

269

whole and noticed its effect on her thoughts or feelings. Anna said that by doing this, she was able to step back and see that there was a bigger picture to what she was experiencing. She saw that her view of the competition was narrow and focused only on having to do well. She also became aware that some of her doubts came from her conflicted feelings about her job and were not necessarily about skating, which she enjoyed.

The breathing space enabled Anna to take an alternative view of some of her more critical thinking. She acknowledged that although the doubtful thoughts might still be with her, she could go out and compete anyway. Anna said that by taking this wider view of what was happening to her, she could see more clearly that her task at this moment was to be at this event and do her best. This allowed her to participate with more enthusiasm and commitment.

Afterwards, it became clear that the breathing space had not just given Anna a pause. It had connected her to the regular formal meditation practice that had become an important aspect of her new daily routine. It was as if, during that short breathing space, Anna had been able to bring to the situation the "wider perspective" she had discovered during her longer, more formal sittings and her work in the classes. She had found particularly helpful the way that formal sitting meditation mixed focusing on the breath with "choiceless awareness" of whatever came up. Choiceless awareness meant that whatever was in moment-to-moment experience could become the object and focus of attention as if it were the breath. The task was to observe anything that arose with bare attention and without judgment. Anna had been surprised at how much meaning could be attached to this moment-by-moment experience, for example, hearing a simple sound. Most of the time, she did not expect sound to carry any emotional overtones whatsoever. Yet for her, listening in this way brought greater awareness of emotions, especially anger and tension. She had also become more aware of how, when tense, her tendency, almost a reflex, was to brace or tighten different parts of her body that had previously escaped her awareness.

The instruction to "open" to such feelings, to "soften" in response to them, allowed Anna to stay with such sensations longer than she might previously have done. The attitude of the instructor had also been important, encouraging her curiosity about such observations, and allowing her to take a wider perspective on experience. She found the instructor's questions became her own. Was this thought or feeling pulling for her attention? What did she notice about this experience? How long did it last? Did it change or stay the same? Was she aware of any thoughts alongside what she was experiencing? How did it fade, if at all? All of this formal practice was now available to her, made present in each situation by her greater awareness of what was going on. Anna's experience when preparing for her competition was that the breathing space was helpful because it was continuous with the rest of her practice, rather than an isolated "quick fix" and a substitute for regular formal practice.

Anna's experience raises an important issue: that it was the sense of "opening" to difficult thoughts, feelings, and sensations that allowed her to see more clearly when she was vulnerable to thinking in old and unproductive ways. She was beginning to identify her own relapse signature. This was one of the important themes for this session, and we turn our attention to it later. First, though, we wanted participants to explore an important option following the breathing space: the action step. To understand why this is important, we return to some theory.

THE IMPORTANCE OF TAKING ACTION IN DEALING WITH DEPRESSION

When we started this project to develop a program to help people prevent depression from coming back, our first thought had been to develop a maintenance version of cognitive-behavioral therapy. Prominent in our plans for such an approach was to focus on teaching people how to notice early signs of impending relapse and then take action to avoid the escalation of mood. As you can now see, the program we eventually adopted contained less cognitive-behavior ther-

BOX 12.1

⊗

Theme and Curriculum for Session 7

THEME

There are some specific things that can be done when depression threatens. Taking a breathing space will come first, and then deciding what action, if any, to take. Each person has his or her own unique warning signs of relapse, but participants can help each other in making plans for how best to respond to the signs.

AGENDA

- 40-minute sitting meditation—awareness of breath, body, sounds, then thoughts (plus noting reactions to introduction of difficulties).
- Practice Review.
- Homework Review (including Series 2 tapes and breathing spaces).
- Exercise to explore links between activity and mood.
- Generate list of pleasure and mastery activities.
- Plan how best to schedule such activities.
- 3-Minute Breathing Space as the "first step" before choosing whether to take mindful action.
- Identifying relapse signatures.
- Identifying actions to deal with threat of relapse/recurrence.
- 3-Minute Breathing Space or mindful walking.
- Distribute Session 6 participant handouts.
- Homework assignment:
  Select, from all the different forms of practice, a pattern you intend to use on a regular basis.
  3-Minute Breathing Space—Regular (three times a day).
  3-Minute Breathing Space—Coping (whenever you notice unpleasant feelings).
  Develop early warning system for detecting relapses.
  Develop action plan to be used in the face of lowered moods.

(cont.)

PREPARATION AND PLANNING

- In addition to your personal preparation, remember to bring a black or white board and writing materials to class for the activity and mood links, relapse signature, and action plan exercises. You will also need a copy of Mary Oliver's poem "The Summer Day."

PARTICIPANT HANDOUTS

Handout 12.1. Summary of Session 7: How Can I Best Take Care of Myself?
Handout 12.2. When Depression Is Overwhelming.
Handout 12.3. Homework for Week Following Session 7.
Handout 12.4. Homework Record Form—Session 7.

---

apy and instead became embedded within a mindfulness-based approach.

But from the outset, we were also concerned that we not lose sight of the fact that cognitive therapy contains many important elements that, together, reduce the chances of relapse. Cognitive-behavior therapy (CBT) is an empirical, action-oriented approach. Its scheduled homework encourages patients to become more aware of the pattern of not only their thinking but also their lives (what they are doing that maintains their depression, what they are not doing that might allow mood to improve). Learning to monitor such daily activities allows patients to notice when their lives begin to get out of control.

But CBT does not stop at monitoring activities: It schedules activities. The theme of "taking action" is all-pervasive in CBT, as a way of either counteracting a period of fatigue or negative mood, or testing the reality of a negative thought, attitude, or belief. We thought it important that MBCT include this element. From time to time, and especially when depression threatens to overwhelm a person, there is a need to explore how activity may help. Such exploration may simply reveal that the amount of activity needs to be increased, or that the quality of activity needs to change.

TAKING CARE OF YOURSELF

It is important to be aware of a major stumbling block for participants in noticing warning signs and taking action. No amount of awareness of the signs of relapse and planning to take action is likely to affect what actually happens to participants unless they are able to learn gradually to take care of themselves and to value the qualities of moment-to-moment experience. (Relatedly, we read Mary Oliver's poem "The Summer Day" during this session; see Box 12.2.) Participants may discover 101 reasons why they do not deserve to take a rest or do things they enjoy, especially when they are feeling down. Recall the CBT approach to this situation. What is imaginative about CBT is that it does not wait until the person feels like doing something before scheduling it to occur. Instead, CBT identifies those actions and activities associated, for each patient, with being non-depressed, and then works collaboratively with the person to build these into the daily routine.

Importantly, cognitive therapists realize that depression reverses the motivation process. Normally, we can wait until we want to do something before we actually do it; in depression, we have to do something before we are able to want to do it. Furthermore, the tiredness and fatigue that occur in depression can be misleading. When we are not depressed, tiredness means that we need to rest. In this case, rest refreshes us. When depressed, however, resting can actually increase tiredness. The fatigue of depression is not normal tiredness; it does not call for rest, but for increased activity, if only for a short while. Part of "taking care" of yourself in those moments is to "stay in the game" or keep participating in activities, even if your mood and thoughts seem to say that there is no use.

Because MBCT was designed for people who are between episodes of depression, it was likely that participants might be able to appreciate the message about "taking care of yourself," if only because they might see the difference between their attitude when depressed and their present attitude, when their mood allowed them to be more evenhanded. Nevertheless, participants felt reluctant to take time for themselves. Actually, this is true for many of us.

BOX 12.2

⚬

"The Summer Day"

Who made the world?
Who made the swan, and the black bear?
Who made the grasshopper?
This grasshopper, I mean—
the one who has flung herself out of the grass,
the one who is eating sugar out of my hand,
who is moving her jaws back and forth instead of up and down—
who is gazing around with her enormous and complicated eyes.
Now she lifts her pale forearms and thoroughly washes her face.
Now she snaps her wings open, and floats away.
I don't know exactly what a prayer is.
I do know how to pay attention, how to fall down
into the grass, how to kneel down in the grass,
how to be idle and blessed, how to stroll through the fields,
which is what I have been doing all day.
Tell me, what else should I have done?
Doesn't everything die at last, and too soon?
Tell me, what is it you plan to do
with your one wild and precious life?

From Mary Oliver, *House of Light*.[79] Copyright 1990 by Mary Oliver. Reprinted by permission of Beacon Press, Boston.

NOTICING THE LINKS BETWEEN ACTIVITY AND MOOD

Take a moment to bring to mind what you do during a typical working day. If you spend much of your day apparently doing the same thing, try breaking the activities down into smaller parts: talking to colleagues, making coffee, filing, word processing, eating lunch. And what about evenings and weekends? What sort of things do you find yourself doing then? Make a list in your mind's eye or on paper. Now see if you can divide the list into (1) those things that lift your mood, give you energy, nourish you; and (2) those things that dampen your mood or drain your energy. Finally, ask yourself how you might be able to find more time to do the things that give you energy, and deal more skillfully with those things that drain you of energy. This exercise is an important component of a CBT approach to depression. It is now time to weave it into MBCT.

Up to this point, the breathing space has involved three steps: (1) acknowledging what is going on in the mind and the body, (2) bringing attention to the breath, and then (3) expanding attention to the body. In the last session, we saw how, following such a breathing space, we might use various means of relating differently to troubling thoughts. We now explore how, following awareness of the breath, taking action is an alternative option.

In order to introduce this option, we ask participants to do the exercise: to write down some of the typical things they do in a day.

When the list is complete, participants categorize the activities into the positive ("What am I doing in my daily life that nourishes me?") and the negative ("What am I doing in my life from day to day that reduces my ability to feel whole, calm, or in the moment?")

Then, in pairs or in small groups participants ask the following questions:

> "Of the positive activities: How might I change things so that I take more time to do these things or become more aware of them?"

> "Of the negative or draining activities: How might these best be done less often?"

The following are some of the comments and observations people have made when doing this exercise in class. One theme that often emerges is a greater awareness of the negative activities that cause problems than of the positive activities. Another common theme is that people often feel guilty if they take time for themselves.

> "There are things in life over which you don't have a choice, like going to work."

> "Most of us are not raised to take time for ourselves."

"You can only do something nice for yourself once your obligations to others, or to your work, have been satisfied."

"I am balancing being a mom, a career woman, a wife, and a housekeeper. Where do I find the time for myself?"

"My parents are elderly and need caring for. It would be wrong for me to put myself first."

"If you don't keep up, you fall behind."

These comments describe how we are all pulled in many directions much of the time. Yet there is another aspect we would do well to notice: They seem to be very general, and to imply that there is no room for things to be different than they are. We can see the impasse here. If we want things to be different, but our thoughts tell us things won't change, then we are stuck. But what if, by becoming more aware of what is happening, we start to "taste the raisin"—to pay more attention even in the midst of the busy-ness. Is there a possibility of "looking for the spaces" even when things are hectic, so that looking after yourself is not an optional extra? Taking action starts with simply noticing what is going on around you.

Take the case of Jackie, a nurse on a busy hospital ward, always, as she said, "being knocked off her feet" with one thing after another. There simply seemed to be no time for her to relax, far less to sit and meditate. But she started to pay more attention within the busy-ness. She noticed that little spaces opened up even at the most hectic times. She said, for example, that she had needed to phone someone in another part of the hospital to get some test results on a patient. She phoned several times but got no reply. This was one of the most frustrating aspects of her job, waiting for someone in another department to answer the phone when she had so much to do. She had started to get angry.

Then, she stopped. Here was 30 seconds in which she could not rush around; here was a moment of potential silence in the noise of the day. She started to use the lack of an answer as an opportunity to take a breathing space, to step back. Gradually, she started to notice many other times when she could step back, for example, pushing a drugs trolley, whose speed limited the pace of movement along the corridor, or walking to the other end of the ward to see a patient's family. Prior to this, she had thought that meditation practice might best be done when taking a lunch break or going to the rest room. Now, she found she could look for the "in-between" spaces throughout the day, spaces that transformed her thoughts, feelings, and behavior for the rest of the activities of the day.

In a way, she had found a way of "turning towards" rather than escaping or avoiding her experience. This is exactly what we ask of each participant: to hold the difficult aspects of their daily lives, as well as their beliefs or expectations about them, and to move closer to them. After all, it is what they have been doing in the practice for the past 6 weeks with bodily sensations, feelings, and thoughts. Having mapped the territory, seeing more clearly what is going on by using the breathing space, it may be time to consider taking action.

ACTION TO TAKE: FOCUSING ON MASTERY AND PLEASURE

We wish to encourage participants to discover how they might best deal with periods of low mood that may lead to depression. The idea is to use day-by-day experience to discover and cultivate activities that can be used as tools to cope with periods of worsening mood. Having these tools already available means that participants will be more likely to persist with them in the face of negative thoughts such as "Why bother with anything?" that are simply part of the territory of depressed mood.

When people feel sad, there are two types of activities that can lift their mood, but that depression tends to undermine. The first type of activity is one that gives pleasure. Once people are depressed, it is harder to enjoy things that they would once have found enjoyable, such as going out for a meal with a friend, taking a nice, long bath, eating dessert, or buying something simply because it would be fun to have it.

The second type of helpful activity that depression undermines is one that gives a sense of mastery. These kinds of activities nourish participants by contributing to a sense of accomplishment, or a feeling that they are "taking care of business." Some of these include writing a letter, filling out an income tax form, shopping for groceries, or mowing the lawn.

Having defined these two types of activity, it is interesting to see what examples the participants can generate from their own experience. Many may seem trivial (e.g., watching a video, phoning a friend). They may have seemed too unimportant to put on the earlier list of things that either nourish or drain energy. But the instruction is to expand the list of "nourishing" activities and put a *P* next to those that give pleasure and an *M* next to those that give a sense of mastery, no matter how trivial. The next stage is to select those activities that might be scheduled in the future. The discussion moves on to how participants can best schedule such activities (including breaking them down into small steps), so that they are not omitted by default.

We give quite specific instructions. When feeling down, first bring awareness to the breath. This is always the first step. Take a breathing space if possible. Then, choose what to do next: either focus on thoughts (see last session) or take action. There is both a general and a specific message here. The general message is that by actually being present in more of our moments, and making mindful decisions about what we really need at each of those moments, we can use activity to become more aware and alert, and to regulate mood. The specific message is that depressed mood cannot be overlooked. We must always make a choice about what (specifically) to do next. This can be expressed simply: In low mood, take a breathing space, then make a choice; be with the thoughts as thoughts, or take action. The nature of depression demands such specificity.

We include in the handouts some hints as to how participants can, after reconnecting with an expanded awareness in the breathing space, move to take some skillful action. As we have seen in dealing with depressed feelings, activities that are pleasurable or give a sense of mastery may be particularly helpful. However, doing things that give pleasure or increase mastery is particularly difficult when mood is low, and the handouts include additional material that participants can read and share with partners or family members outside the class. Whatever action is taken, the idea is to act mindfully: to ask, "What do I need for myself right now? How can I best take care of myself right now?"

SOME TIPS ABOUT TAKING ACTION WHEN YOUR MOOD IS LOW

Some people have found the following "tips" are useful in keeping perspective on what activity can or cannot do for them:

- As best you can, perform your action as an experiment, without prejudging how you will feel after it is completed. Keep an open mind about whether doing this will be helpful in any way.
- Consider a range of activities and don't limit yourself to a favorite few. Sometimes, trying new behaviors can be interesting in itself. "Exploring" and "inquiring" often work to diminish "withdrawal" and "retreat" reactions.
- Don't expect miracles. Try to carry out what you have planned as best you can. Putting extra pressure on yourself by expecting your new approach to alter things dramatically may be unrealistic. Rather, activities are helpful in building your overall sense of control in the face of shifts in your mood. They are also helpful in allowing you to see how the practice of mindfulness can influence your behavior.

IDENTIFYING THE RELAPSE SIGNATURES

The research we reviewed in Chapter 3 showed that when people have been depressed many times, the process of becoming depressed can become more and more autonomous. The depression gathers pace very fast and seems to escalate without external triggers. This means that it is important to identify in advance, and while mood is stable, those changes (in mind and body) that might signal that depression is developing. By being able to recognize these signs early, participants will be in a better position to use the skills that they have been practicing. These signs of relapse, referred to as "relapse signatures," are unique for each individual.

Note that this assumes an acceptance that depression will occur again, but we are working with how to handle or deal with it when it occurs. It would be a mistake to think that taking a mindfulness class means that you might never feel sadness again. It is rather a question of learning better how to take care of ourselves when it happens, charting the territory of depression, so that we can navigate through it with less fear.

We examine relapse signatures by setting an exercise for the class that is best started in pairs or small groups. The task is to make a list of the specific warning signals that depression might be trying to take hold again. Once finished, the instructor writes some of the signals on the blackboard, including the following:

- Becoming irritable,
- Decreasing social participation—just "not wanting to see people"
- Changing sleep habits
- Changing eating habits
- Getting easily exhausted
- Giving up on exercise
- Not wanting to deal with business (opening mail, paying bills, etc.)
- Postponing deadlines

Each person's particular combination of signs of impending relapse or recurrence is unique. Becoming aware without becoming hypervigilant for these signs is an important balance to discover. But just noticing these changes isn't enough. It is easy to list them when we are feeling good, but when our mood starts to worsen, we may no longer believe that it is useful to heed these warnings at all. Recall that part of the "territory" of depression is hopelessness. And hopelessness tends to make us feel that none of these practices is worth doing, that "I am back to square one." That is why participants are encouraged to take advantage of their present intention to look after themselves and include others in their plans. They need to ask themselves two questions: "What, in the past, has prevented me from noticing and attending to these feelings (e.g., pushing away, denial, distraction, self-medication with alcohol; arguments, blaming family members or colleagues)?" and "How can I include other family members in my early warning system for detecting the signs of a relapse?"

ACTION PLAN TO DEAL WITH THREAT OF RELAPSE/RECURRENCE

Participants return to their pairs or small groups to discuss action plans and to see what sort of strategies they might adopt.

- The first step is always to take a breathing space.
- The second step is for participants to make a choice, using other practices that they have found helpful in the past to gather themselves as best they can (e.g., putting on a mindfulness practice tape; reminding themselves what they learned in the class; determining what they found helpful then; going back to something they read or heard during class that captured the essential message of the program; reminding themselves that the feelings are very intense right now, but what they need now is no different from what they practiced then).
- The third step is to take some action, especially action that in the past would have given a sense of pleasure or mastery, even if it seems futile to do so right now (see participant handouts). Break activities down into smaller parts (e.g., deciding to do only part of a task, or restricting themselves to doing it for only a short and easily manageable period of time).

The important thing is to let the past experience of relapse be the teacher. Some participants decide to write themselves a letter, listing five things they like about themselves and consider to be true. Then, they describe some of the ways they might try to talk themselves out of believing this, if they start to feel sad, including the idea that the letter is just a gimmick! They include a list of actions to take, with an instruction to choose at least one, even if they expect not to feel like doing it at the time. Then, they seal the letter and open it only when they start to feel depressed. This, they decide, is the best way to give themselves the benefit of the hard-earned wisdom that might not be available to them at the time.

Participants report that the worst times are often when depression comes out of the blue, for example, on waking up in the morning. We encourage them to start by taking a breathing space. At these times, it is also important to ask themselves: "How can I best be kind to myself right now? What is the best gift I can give to myself at this moment?" Asking specific questions is helpful: "I may not know how long this mood will last; how can I best look after myself until it passes?" Given that the negative thinking can be quite overwhelming in such situations, participants have the chance to observe the tendency of the mind at these moments to be drawn into rumination ("Why am I feeling like this?", "What's wrong with me?", "I should be better than this," "A good parent would feel more energetic about getting their children ready for school; this means I am a bad parent"). If they choose to deal with the mood at that moment (rather than the alternative option of dealing with it later), participants report that it is more helpful to ask how the mood is affecting the body, and to bring awareness to the bodily sensations, in order to "open" and "soften." Then they find it easier to make an intentional choice about what to do next.

What we are saying here is that when things are tough, the task is really to focus on each moment, to "handle each moment as best you can." If the quality with which a person handles a difficult moment shifts even by 1%, then that is an important shift, because it affects the next moment, and the next, and so on; so one small change can have a large impact in the end.

USING HOMEWORK TO PREPARE FOR THE END OF THE CLASSES

Given that this will be the last homework to be assigned, it is important for participants to continue to develop routines for practicing on their own (we return to this theme again in Session 8 to remind people of the importance of regular practice). We ask them to spend some quality time between now and the next session making concrete plans for relapse prevention.

We ask them to choose from among all the different types of formal mindfulness practice they have experienced (Series 1 and 2 tapes, combined tape, mindfulness of breath/body without tape, etc.) a form of practice on which they intend to settle on a regular, daily basis for the next few weeks (or until the first follow-up meeting of the class). Having chosen, their instructions are to use this practice on a daily basis this week and record reactions on the Homework Record Form.

In addition to the 3-Minute Breathing Space, participants are given instructions about how to add an action step to it, whenever they notice unpleasant thoughts or feelings (see participant handouts for details).

Finally, there are instructions in the participant handouts for how to involve family members in the task of detecting relapse. The task we give participants is to write down suggestions for an action plan that might be used as a framework for coping action, once they or their friends or family notice early warning signs. They are reminded to address the frame of mind in which they will be at the time (e.g., "I know you probably will not be keen on this idea but I think that, nonetheless, it is very important that you . . . "). For example, they might put on a yoga, body scan, or mindfulness tape; remind themselves what they learned during the class, what was helpful then; take frequent breathing spaces leading into thought review or considered action (appropriately broken down into simple steps, if necessary); read something that would "reconnect" with their "wiser" mind; and so on. It is important that instructors review these ideas during the next, final class.

⊗

Summary of Session 7:
How Can I Best Take Care of Myself

What we actually *do* with our time from moment to moment, from hour to hour, from one year to the next, can be a very powerful influence affecting our general well-being and our ability to deal skillfully with depression.

You might like to try asking yourself these questions:

1. Of the things that I do, what nourishes me, what increases my sense of actually being alive and present rather than merely existing? (up activities)

2. Of the things that I do, what drains me, what decreases my sense of actually being alive and present, what makes me feel I am merely existing, or worse? (down activities)

3. Accepting that there are some aspects of my life that I simply cannot change, am I consciously choosing to increase the time and effort I give to up activities and to decrease the time and effort I give to down activities?

By being actually present in more of our moments and making mindful decisions about what we really need in each of those moments, we can use activity to become more aware and alert, and to regulate mood.

This is true for dealing with both the regular pattern of our daily lives and periods of low mood that may lead to depression—we can use our day-by-day experience to discover and cultivate activities that we can use as tools to cope with periods of worsening mood. Having these tools already available means that we will be more likely to persist with them in the face of negative thoughts such as "Why bother with anything?" that are simply part of the territory of depressed mood.

For example, one of the simplest ways to take care of your physical and mental well-being is to take daily physical exercise—as a minimum, aim for three brisk, 10-minute walks a day and also, if at all possible, other types of exercise, such as mindful stretching, yoga, swimming, jogging, and so on. Once exercise is in your daily routine, it is a readily available response to depressed moods as they arise.

The breathing space provides a way to remind us to use activity to deal with unpleasant feelings as they arise.

(cont.)

USING THE BREATHING SPACE: THE ACTION STEP

After reconnecting with an expanded awareness in the breathing space, it may feel appropriate to take some *considered action*. In dealing with depressed feelings, the following activities may be particularly helpful:

1. Do something pleasurable.
2. Do something that will give you a sense of satisfaction or mastery.
3. Act mindfully.

Ask yourself: What do I need for myself right now? How can I best take care of myself right now?

Try some of the following:

1. Do something pleasurable.

   Be kind to your body: Have a nice hot bath; have a nap; treat yourself to your favorite food without feeling guilty; have your favorite hot drink; give yourself a facial or manicure.

   Engage in enjoyable activities: Go for a walk (maybe with the dog or a friend); visit a friend; do your favorite hobby; do some gardening; take some exercise; phone a friend; spend time with someone you like; cook a meal; go shopping; watch something funny or uplifting on TV; read something that gives you pleasure; listen to music that makes you feel good.

2. Do something that gives you a sense of mastery, satisfaction, achievement, or control.

   Clean the house; clear out a cupboard or drawer; catch up with letter writing; do some work; pay a bill; do something that you have been putting off doing; take some exercise (N.B. It's especially important to congratulate yourself whenever you complete a task or part of a task *and to break tasks down into smaller steps and only tackle one step at a time.*)

3. Act mindfully (read Staying Present, Handout 9.4).

   Focus your entire attention on just what you are doing right now; keep yourself in the very moment you are in; put your mind in the present (e.g., "Now I am walking down the stairs ... now I can feel the banister beneath my hand ... now I'm walking into the kitchen ... now I'm turning on the light ... "); be aware of your breathing as you do other things; be aware of the contact of your feet with the floor as you walk.

(cont.)

REMEMBER

1. Try to perform your action as an experiment. Try not to prejudge how you will feel after it is completed. Keep an open mind about whether doing this will be helpful in any way.
2. Consider a range of activities and don't limit yourself to a favorite few. Sometimes, trying new behaviors can be interesting in itself. "Exploring" and "inquiring" often work against "withdrawal" and "retreat."
3. Don't expect miracles. Try to carry out what you have planned as best you can. Putting extra pressure on yourself by expecting this to alter things dramatically may be unrealistic. Rather, activities are helpful in building your overall sense of control in the face of shifts in your mood.

⊗⊗

When Depression Is Overwhelming

Sometimes you may find that depression comes out of the blue. For example, you may wake up feeling very tired and listless, with hopeless thoughts going through your mind.

When this happens, it may be useful for you to tell yourself, *"Just because I am depressed now does not mean that I have to stay depressed."*

When things come out of the blue like this, they set off negative ways of thinking in everyone.

If you have been depressed in the past, it will tend to trigger old habits of thought that may be particularly damaging: full of overgeneralizations, predictions that this will go on forever, and "back to square one" thinking. All of these ways of making sense of what is happening to you will tend to undermine your taking any action.

Having these symptoms does not mean that it needs to go on for a long time or that you are already in a full-blown episode of depression.

Ask yourself, "What can I do to look after myself to get me through this low period?"

Take a breathing space to help gather yourself. This may help you see your situation from a wider perspective. This wider perspective allows you to become aware of both the pull of the old habits of thinking and what skillful action you might take.

⊗
Homework for Week Following Session 7

1. From all the different forms of formal mindfulness practice you have experienced (Series 1 and 2 tapes, combined tape, mindfulness of breath/body without tape, etc.), settle on a form of practice that you intend to use on a regular, daily basis for the next 5 weeks. Use this practice on a daily basis this week, and record your reactions on the Homework Record Form.
2. 3-Minute Breathing Space—Regular: Practice three times a day at times that you have decided in advance. Record each time you do it by circling an *R* for the appropriate day on the Homework Record Form; note any comments/difficulties.
3. 3-Minute Breathing Space—Coping plus Action: Practice *whenever you notice unpleasant thoughts or feelings*. Record each time you do the coping breathing space by circling an *X* for the appropriate day on the Homework Record Form; note any comments/difficulties.

RELAPSE PREVENTION

What are your warning signals that depression might be trying to take hold again (e.g., becoming irritable; decreased social contact—just "not wanting to see people"; changes in sleeping habits; changes in eating habits; getting easily exhausted; giving up on exercise; not wanting to deal with business such as opening mail, paying bills, etc.; postponing deadlines)?

Set up an Early Warning System—write down on the next blank sheet the changes that you should look out for (if it feels comfortable, include *those with whom you share your life* in a collaborative effort to *notice* and then to *respond* rather than to *react* to these signs).

Write down on the next blank sheet suggestions to yourself for an Action Plan that you can use as a framework for coping action, once you or your friends/family have noticed early warning signs (remember to address the frame of mind that you will be in at the time, e.g., "I know you probably will not be keen on this idea but I think that, nonetheless, it is very important that you ... "). For example, you might put on a yoga, body scan, or mindfulness tape; remind yourself of what you learned during the class that was helpful then; take frequent breathing spaces leading into thought review or considered action; read something that will "reconnect" you with your "wiser" mind, and so on.

It may be helpful to remind yourself that what you need at times of difficulty is no different from what you have already practiced many times throughout this course.

Name: _____

Record on the Homework Record Form each time you practice. Also, make a note of anything that comes up in the homework, so that we can talk about it at the next meeting.

Day/date	Practice (Yes/No)	Comments
Wednesday Date:	Tape: R R R × × × × × × × × × × ×	
Thursday Date:	Tape: R R R × × × × × × × × × × ×	
Friday Date:	Tape: R R R × × × × × × × × × × ×	
Saturday Date:	Tape: R R R × × × × × × × × × × ×	
Sunday Date:	Tape: R R R × × × × × × × × × × ×	
Monday Date:	Tape: R R R × × × × × × × × × × ×	
Tuesday Date:	Tape: R R R × × × × × × × × × × ×	
Wednesday Date:	Tape: R R R × × × × × × × × × × ×	

CHAPTER 13

⊗

Using What Has Been Learned to Deal with Future Moods

SESSION 8

If there were a way to pull together the central ideas covered in the course, what would it be? Perhaps it is this: that when relapse-related automatic thought patterns are triggered, there are skillful ways of responding to them. These ways do not deny that there is a problem with which people must deal. But they remind people that there are choices, one of which is to face whatever is causing the depression, and the depression itself, in a radically different way. Instead of ruminating about the problem; instead of asking unanswerable questions such as "Why me" and "What is it about me that causes this?", instead of the thoughts of failure that just go around in circles, there exists another possibility.

The task becomes that of holding whatever thoughts, feelings, or sensations we become aware of in mindfulness along with the breath. As we have seen before, we never know what we might find! In due course, people may come to understand, and to experience at a very deep level, that the mind has a way of processing the "stuff of every-day life" in a way that is wiser than they might have imagined. Learning to trust that this process will occur without interference from other, more problem-solving modes of mind is difficult.

Using a computer analogy may help. Many people buy comput-ers to do relatively simple tasks such as word processing or tracking accounts. We are now told that much of the computing power on an average desktop PC is never called upon to perform. Now, imagine that the situation with our minds is something similar: that we have a "processor" in our minds (the "Great Computer Within") that can, if allowed to do so, help process the difficulties and problems that accu-mulate during our lifetimes; that the reason for allowing it to do so is because it is able to handle things in a much wiser and gentler way than we ever could do normally; that this different mode of mind is always available to us, though the busy-ness of our lives often ob-scures it.

Whether or not we find this analogy helpful, it remains true that not all situations call for action or efforts to make changes. In the realm of emotions, things often don't follow logically. It might be that in some areas of our lives, the harder we try, the more we can achieve. But this rule seldom applies when we are dealing with feel-ings that we don't want to have or aspects of ourselves of which we are critical.

It may be a paradox, but *if we cope with our unpleasant feelings by pushing them away or trying to control them, we actually end up maintaining them.* This is the last thing we would expect; yet it re-mains true. In avoiding or "pushing away" our experience, we remain limited in understanding its wider context. Yet as soon as we accept that we feel sad or anxious, in that moment, it is already different. Ac-cepting that we feel a certain way doesn't mean that we have to ap-prove of it, nor does it mean that we are finally defeated by it and might just as well give up. Quite the contrary, by accepting how we feel, we are just telling ourselves that this is our starting point. We are actually in a better position to decide what to do.

Of course, the ability to decide which course to take—whether to act to bring about change or to accept how things are for now—will depend on many things, not least of which is our momentary awareness of what is called for in any situation. *Sometimes wisdom means not to act.*

It might be that our situation is genuinely difficult or chaotic. If so, we may need simply to "be with" the sense of difficulty or chaos, allowing ourselves to take a good look at it. This looking might bring up a sense of uncertainty, and if so, some anxiety. But if we can allow uncertainty to be here, resisting the temptation to act just because we can't stand the uncertainty, then there is a much greater chance that we will see things clearly. If we can experience the chaos and uncertainty consciously, the chaos itself can take us to the clarity. And if we need a brake on the mind's tendency to want to act impulsively, its tendency to prefer any course of action to the anguish that accompanies confusion, then we can always come back to the breath.

LOOKING BACK

This being the last session, we look back to what participants have learned. As in MBSR, we start this last session by first using the body scan as the formal practice, to give a sense of coming full circle. Second, we make time for participants to recall their experiences over the period of the program, scheduling an exercise to allow people to think back. While the last class together naturally brings to mind thoughts of endings and partings, there is a way in which Session 8 is more like the end of the beginning rather than the beginning of the end. Because what is being asked is not bounded by time limits or deadlines, "the real Session 8", as Jon Kabat-Zinn has said, "is the rest of our lives."

It is interesting to hear how people respond to the body scan now that they have come to the end of the classes. With a greater sense of how attention can be trained and reclaimed, the body scan is viewed by most in a different way than it was 8 weeks earlier. This does not mean that participants have all fallen in love with it. In fact, those who found parts of it boring or tedious still often say that this was the case. What is new, however, is that when people find it boring, it bothers them less. They are better able to recognize that even this "negative" experience can teach them about being with boredom

BOX 13.1

⊗

Theme and Curriculum for Session 8

THEME

Maintaining a balance in life is helped by regular mindfulness practice. Good intentions can be strengthened by linking such intentions to a positive reason for taking care of oneself.

AGENDA

- Body Scan Practice.
- Practice Review.
- Homework Review (including early warning systems and action plans).
- Review whole course: what has been learned—in pairs, then go around whole group.
- Give out questionnaire for participants to give personal reflections on the program.
- Discuss how best to keep up momentum and discipline developed over the past 7 weeks in both formal and informal practice.
- Check and discuss plans, and link them to positive reasons for maintaining the practice.
- Distribute Session 8 participant handouts.
- End the classes with a concluding meditation (marble, stone, or bead).

PREPARATION AND PLANNING

In addition to your personal preparation, remember to bring the Session 8 questionnaire. A black or white board may be helpful to record participants' choices for maintaining practice and relapse prevention plans. Also, remember to bring a memento for each participant, to mark the end of the program.

PARTICIPANT HANDOUTS

Handout 13.1. Summary of Session 8: Using What Has Been Learned to Deal with Future Moods.
Handout 13.2. Daily Mindfulness.

or tedium, if that is what they are experiencing. Others in the class remember the body scan as very helpful to them, and, when the homework has given them the opportunity, have returned to it in some form. For them, the opportunity to do the body scan again in the class is an affirmation of their practice with it over the past 7 weeks. Following the feedback on the practice, we set time aside for people to look back.

"Looking back now, I can see. . . . " The instruction is to spend some time, alone or in pairs, reflecting on a number of questions:

- "Think back to why you came originally—what were your expectations and why did you stay?"
- "What did you want/hope for?"
- "What did you get out of coming, if anything? What did you learn?"
- "What were the costs to you?"
- "What are your biggest blocks/obstacles to continuing?"
- "What strategies might help you not get stuck?"

In addition to this exercise, participants spend a few minutes writing down their personal reflections about the program. We use a simple questionnaire that asks people to say, on a scale from 1 to 10 (1, "not at all important," and 10, "extremely important"), how important the program has been to them. We then leave the page blank and say to them, "Please say why you have given it this rating."

It is perhaps inevitable that we, as instructors, new to a mindfulness approach, are intrigued to hear what participants got out of the course. Reading these comments after the program was over, it was impossible not to be struck by the commonalities in the participants' experience: It had been hard, but it had been a challenge worth accepting.

"It has given me the opportunity to learn how to give myself space for slowing down and *being*—especially being in the moment. I know that I have a safe place—an inner, safe place that allows me to be me, without any hassles, criticisms, and so on, from other people—and learning to give it priority (the space, that is) on a regular basis helps defuse negative mental thoughts before they cause any more damage."

"This program has confirmed and repeated some things I already knew about depression—but it has been more effective to be able to go through it with other people who know what it's like."

"The good and the not so good—it is a tremendous beginning for me to learn about myself and accept all thoughts and feelings. The breath has been unexpectedly rewarding."

"I have discovered an inner strength."

"I now have tactics when I sense a low mood/depression starting."

"It has removed a sense of shame about having been depressed and anxious in the past, therefore greater self-acceptance."

"I have discovered a way of moving into an inner place of calm/ centeredness."

"My depression and associated anxiety had made me very unhappy. . . . I have been able to actually enjoy and be in the present moment . . . realizing this is the only time I have to live . . . so instead of constantly worrying about the future and my past failures, I can more evenly and calmly embrace the present moment. This has allowed me to realize what it is that makes me depressed . . . and how I can recognize these factors to hopefully alleviate any relapse."

"The meditation brought up a lot of strange emotions that worried me at first, but now I realize that they were just emotions that I had been repressing for years and that to really live my life, I had to feel them. Although I may get down again at times, my whole perspective on life has changed."

These statements are representative of the immediate responses given during Session 8 of the program and written down when the instructor was nearby. It is always possible that, under these circumstances, participants might wish to speak more of the benefits and less of any difficulties. It is interesting, therefore, to see what participants said some months later, when our colleague, Oliver Mason, interviewed them. Listen to one participant as he looks back over the classes. We pick up the interview as he is discussing his early experience with the formal practice.

P: I did the body scan every day, and like every body else, found it relaxing, perhaps too relaxing. But that had its benefits, too, because one of the things when you are depressed is this difficulty in relaxing and finding sleep, finding recuperation. You seem to have this motor that's overrunning all the time inside you. So something that can give you that deep relaxation was and is quite valuable. But the rest of the tapes, I did what I was supposed to do.

Interviewer: So you went through the course as it was presented to you. Any discoveries or surprises that stick out?

P: The key thing overall has been that often what goes through your mind are just mental phenomena. They are just thoughts, they are just that, they are just thoughts, not necessarily truths. And you do have some choice about which ones to follow. I mean, I am not saying it's necessarily easy to do that. But that idea I found very, very helpful: that you are not a victim of thoughts going on in your mind, a sort of helpless victim just bobbing along with them. You can choose to disregard some and look at others more closely, and look at why those are cropping up more often and with more insistence.

The participant goes on to describe how he is now more able to bring a wider, decentered view to his thoughts and feelings.

Interviewer: And you are not quite so close to the problem, either? It's there but you are not it?

P: Yes, exactly. It's not just happening to you; you can see it happening to you. There is a very very big difference there, I think. And I've always felt the biggest challenge comes when you are feeling pretty low. Because at those times, it is less easy to meditate. I find there's less motivation to do it, but the need to do it is greater. I suppose at good times I tend not to do so much formal meditation, but when things are bad, it's important to do it, I think, because it reconnects you to the whole program and the whole ethos behind it, which you can easily forget, you know, if you just start to go down.

This raises the issues that were discussed in Session 7: how do people recognize their relapse signatures?

Interviewer: So how do you spot that, when you start to go down?

P: For me, I think the triggers are sluggishness, disturbed sleep, waking up at all times of the night, futility, and hopelessness about things. Not dramatic, but a lowering of your morale and a sort of physical slowness or weakness pervading things.

Interviewer: So does that bring you back to meditating straightway?

P: Not straightaway, at least not always. It's a prompt to do something, certainly. I don't always honor that. I don't always respond to that prompt. But before the program, I would have simply been dragged along, dragged down by it, and I would have felt more hopeless, like there were no kind of support or props, there was no way other than taking pills.

Interviewer: So it's a sense that there is at least something you can do?

P: Yes, it doesn't promise to cure depression, but it's a strategy for dealing with it, which gives you some control over what is happening to you. I suppose that is the key of it, really.

This participant appears to feel differently about his depression. By knowing what the signs of impending depression are for him, and seeing them as prompts, he is able to talk about having choices. He admits how easy it is to forget the program when he feels his mood lowering but is able to use the practice to "reconnect to the whole program." Fundamentally, his relationship to his thoughts has altered. ". . . what goes through your mind are just mental phenomena. They are just thoughts, they are just that, they are just thoughts, not necessarily truths. And you do have some choice about which ones to follow." He appears to have a spirit of discovery about his moods and his thoughts. Finally, he has no illusions about the future, nor about a "cure" for his depression.

His experience was that, even months after the classes had finished, he felt able to deal with upsetting events in a way that did not trigger the severe depression that, he felt, would have occurred before. For him, the program appeared to have prevented recurrence of major depression. His experience raises important issues: first, how to keep the practice alive once the classes have ended, and second, how to deal effectively and skillfully with future downturns in mood.

LOOKING FORWARD

Finding a way to set up and maintain practice in the absence of weekly classes is a challenge faced by all participants. It is important to set time aside to hear what type of practice people have decided they will settle on. Because there are a number of choices, the plans are quite varied. Sometimes we find it helpful to list them on the blackboard. Some participants say that they will continue to practice for 30 minutes on a regular basis. Others report that they will alternate between a regular sitting practice and yoga. More usually, participants say that they do not know whether they can sustain the same level of practice they achieved during the course. Instead, they aim to use the breathing space throughout the day and then practice more formally on the weekend or when they feel the need to "refresh" their practice. Others have found one of the tapes from Series 2 particularly helpful. For example, the mountain meditation has enabled many of them to explore how to relate to patterns of negative thoughts and feelings as if these were storms blowing around the top of a mountain. For still others, a tape that simply contains the sound of bells ringing occasionally gives them sufficient structure to sit without instructions. Whatever the proposed plan the important thing is that it should be realistic.

Occasionally, the question arises: Is it OK just to sit on the weekends, if one sits long enough? It is important for instructors to be sensitive about giving choices and instruction. Of course, the choice is up to participants, but experience shows that regular, daily, brief practice is preferable to longer but infrequent practice. There is something about the "everydayness" of the practice (no matter how short) that is important. Continuity builds, and sustains motivation and momentum. Because relating to our experience mindfully is not part of the territory of the depressed mind, we need all the help we can get in connecting back to it. People need whatever support they can give themselves, whether it is a favorite tape, special quotes, or any other reminders. It is like learning a foreign language: It is better to keep speaking it at every opportunity and on a regular basis.

One of the main reasons instructors devote so much time to this topic has to do with the fact that stress is unpredictable. Nobody knows when and where depression will hit. Yet we also know from studies of cognitive therapy that the people who benefit most from the treatment are those who do the homework. If people can manage to keep the practice fresh, keeping it there each day, each week, then it is much more available than if they let it go. We need to keep our tools oiled, so that they are ready for use when we actually need them.

RELAPSE PREVENTION ACTION PLANS

And what of participants' relapse prevention action plans? These were discussed in Session 7. Participants were to develop such plans during the week for homework. The idea was that if people had an early warning system in place and had written down some helpful things to do, they could draw on these in times of need. Participants discussed a number of these ideas, many of which were based on their experience of *not* having a plan like this available the last time they became depressed.

Liz, a woman in her mid-30s, who felt that the classes had taught her about the need to anticipate how to respond to her changing moods, suggested that she was going to make a list and call it "My Antidepressant Activity List," and file it away until she needed to consult it. For her, this list would include material from the participant handouts, with instructions to herself saying, "Although you may not feel like doing any of these, select at least one and do it anyway":

- Do something today just because you enjoy it.
  - Phone a friend.
  - Rent a video you enjoy.
  - Have a nice, hot bath.
  - Have a nap.
  - Treat yourself to your favorite food, without feeling guilty.
  - Have your favorite hot drink.
  - Go for a walk (maybe with the dog or a friend).
  - Visit a friend.
  - Do your favorite hobby.
  - Spend time with someone you like.
  - Cook a meal.
  - Go shopping.
  - Watch something funny or uplifting on television.
  - Read something that gives you pleasure.
  - Listen to music that makes you feel good.

- Do something that gives you a sense of mastery, satisfaction, achievement, or control.
  - Clean the house.
  - Clear out a cupboard or drawer.
  - Catch up with letter writing.
  - Do some work.
  - Pay a bill.
  - Do some gardening.
  - Do something that you have been putting off doing.
  - Take some exercise.

- Remember to take that big task and break it down into smaller steps (e.g., just do 10 minutes of it) and to congratulate yourself afterwards.

There can be many such ideas floating around. The important thing is to emphasize that any of these might be used in tandem with an early warning system, so long as people decide to do something early enough in the process.

GIVING ONESELF A REASON FOR KEEPING UP THE PRACTICE

Our experience has shown that no matter how good these resolutions are, unless they are linked to a positive reason to do them, they are very difficult to adopt. We find it helpful, therefore, to ask each participant to think of one positive reason for maintaining the practice and having relapse prevention strategies in place. The idea is to link the maintenance of practice with something about which they care deeply.

For example, one participant, Joanne, said that during the classes, she found that she seemed to have more time for her children, that she felt more "available" to them and enjoyed them more. This, she felt, was ironic given that, earlier on in the program, she had been very concerned that the formal practice was taking time away from her children and her husband. She was able to link the plan to maintain some form of everyday practice with her wish to remain available for her children.

At base there is, in a sense, one core reason for maintaining the practice and having relapse prevention strategies in place: "Because I care for myself." Of course, taking care of oneself is *the* problem in depression. What was it that Joanne was discovering?

In the Welsh language, there is a word *trugaredd*, which comes from the root word *caru*, meaning "to love." But because it includes a sense of kindness and unfailing affection, it is often translated "mercy," or "loving-kindness." Depression brings with it the opposite of *trugaredd*: attitudes of self-criticism, self-denigration, and even self-loathing. It undermines the motivation to be kind to oneself and, with it, the capacity to be available to others. The mindfulness approach invites people to explore a different way in which they may relate to themselves and their world, with a quality of attention that has something of *trugaredd* about it. *Trugaredd*, loving-kindness, never works in one direction only. What Joanne had found, to her surprise, was that if she took care of herself, she became more available to others.

These may seem like impossible goals, but we are not talking about striving for goals. We are instead speaking of having an intention: to continue exploring how to become more aware of "where we are" from moment to moment; to explore how to step into "being" mode rather than remain in "doing" mode. This involves practicing mindfulness throughout the day. Here are Larry Rosenberg's tips[71] (pp. 168–170) for how this is done:

1. When possible, do just one thing at a time.
2. Pay full attention to what you are doing.
3. When the mind wanders from what you are doing, bring it back.
4. Repeat Step 3 several billion times.
5. Investigate your distractions.

THE POWER IN THE SIMPLICITY

What we have found remarkable is that the program has effects on participants without ever being part of the "agenda" of the sessions. In particular, the mindfulness practice seems to allow the wider perspective, which has been learned in relation to ordinary daily events, to generalize in unexpected ways. Listen to the following account of someone looking back on the difference it made to practice mindfulness, first in dealing with the humdrum routine of each day, and then in coping at a very difficult period of his life, when his father died.

P: This morning, for instance, is a case in point. I had a lot of things
to do this morning as usual. It's Monday morning, the dustbin
had to go out, and I only had about half an hour to do these
things, and I found myself, oh God, I reached the point when I
stopped and I couldn't go in any direction. It's as if I had gone totally into mind overload. And I thought, "Oh, hang on." And it's
as if there is a switch in the mind now that goes: "Hang on, stop.
Be mindful, and we will start with this bit first." It's like an automatic correction. Instead of getting bogged down with the mind,
trying to do a whole lot of stuff up front, as it were, and overload
me . . . it's the ability to step back from that and hold the mind
there. Just sort it out, as it were, just do one thing. I think that is
the thing that it does. It gives focus all the time. Because it is
easy to be swamped by whatever's on the mind.

Interviewer: And that ability remains even in periods of lowness?

P: It does, yes. I don't know what it does. It's so powerful, yet it is
so simple. . . . And I can go to that point through mindfulness or
meditation and hold or be with whatever happens. If I get low,
for instance, or like I lost my father last year, so there was a lot of
grief. And I was able to meditate with that grief and actually see
it or feel it come up and allow it to come out. Because one of the
problems I had was bottling things up. So I feel myself getting
unhappy about losing my father, so I'm able to sit quietly, allow it
come up and have a good cry. Before, I wouldn't have been able
to cry, it was just a pain here. So that's just being able to sit and
just to watch the thing come up, so that's one of the things it
does. . . . It's been a very valuable grief and a very honest and
pure one, and I find now, when I think of my father, there is less
of a sense of loss and grief and more of a sense of honoring him,
so its been good in that respect. Though I still miss him, it is a
different thing.

Notice what happened here. At no point in the program had
we dealt with his responses to loss or bereavement in the past, or
the vulnerable attitudes he might have had that made it difficult for

him to cope with strong emotions. Yet his experience was that something fundamental had changed for him. Recall that, at the outset, we had wanted to develop an approach that might be used with people who were vulnerable to depression, but who were OK at the moment. We had chosen to explore mindfulness because, among other things, it seemed to provide a way in which people might use the moment-by-moment events of everyday life to learn things that would help them respond to the more difficult events and more severe moods. This participant's experience suggests that, for him, this approach had done just that. Like the participant whose comments we read earlier, MBCT appeared to help him deal with events in his life in a way that helped to prevent a recurrence of major depression. The question remained whether this "preventive" effect would occur in enough participants for us to be confident that these comments were not just isolated incidents. It was a question we would not be able to answer until we had done the necessary statistical evaluation of the whole program, and we come to this issue in Chapter 14.

ENDING THE CLASS

How should the last class end? Simply saying "good-bye and good luck" seems rather weak. People naturally feel they want to remember each other, to wish each other well. So we arranged to give each participant a small object, such as a marble, stone, or bead, and led the class in a short meditation in which they examined the object as we examined the raisin in the first session. The object is a reminder to participants that they have been in the class, a reminder of the hard work they have done over the past 8 weeks, and of the people that have shared this experience with them. And, above all, it is a reminder for participants to continue the process they started, to discover a way of living alongside the damaged aspects of themselves, and to hold before them the possibility of responding to their own fragility in an ever more gentle and more caring way.

⊗

Summary of Session 8—Using What Has Been Learned to Deal with Future Moods

The advantages of awareness, acceptance, and mindfully *responding* to situations rather than immediately running off preprogrammed, "automatic" *reactions* has been a recurring theme throughout this course.

Acceptance may often be the springboard to some form of skillful action directed at achieving change in participants' inner or outer worlds. However, there are also situations and feelings that it may be very difficult, or actually impossible, to change. In this situation, there is the danger that, by carrying on, trying to solve an insoluble problem, or by refusing to accept the reality of the situation one is in, one may end up "banging one's head on a brick wall," exhausting oneself, and actually increasing one's sense of helplessness and depression. In these situations, *you can still retain some sense of dignity and control by making a conscious, mindful, decision not to attempt to exert control and to accept the situation as it is, if possible, with a kindly attitude to the situation and your reactions to it. Choosing* not to act is much less likely to increase depression than being forced to give up attempts at control after repeated failures.

In the so-called "Serenity Prayer," we ask for the *grace to accept with serenity the things that cannot be changed, the courage to change the things that should be changed, and the wisdom to distinguish one from the other.*

Where do we find this grace, this courage, this wisdom? At some level, we *already* have all of these qualities—our task is to realize them (make them real), and our way is none other than moment-by-moment mindful awareness.

THE FUTURE

Remember Jon Kabat-Zinn's advice to weave your parachute every day, rather than leave it to the time you have to jump from the plane!

Decide, right now, what your regular pattern of practice will be over the next weeks, until we meet again, and stick to it as best you can throughout this period. Note any difficulties that you have, so that we can discuss them next time.

Also, remember that the regular breathing space practice provides a way of "checking in with yourself" a few times a day. Let it also be your first response in times of difficulty, stress, or unhappiness—KEEP BREATHING!

☆

Daily Mindfulness

- When you first wake up in the morning, before you get out of bed, bring your attention to your breathing. Observe five mindful breaths.
- Notice changes in your posture. Be aware of how your body and mind feel when you move from lying down to sitting, to standing, to walking. Notice each time you make a transition from one posture to the next.
- Whenever you hear a phone ring, a bird sing, a train pass by, laughter, a car horn, the wind, the sound of a door closing—use any sound as the bell of mindfulness. Really listen and be present and awake.
- Throughout the day, take a few moments to bring your attention to your breathing. Observe five mindful breaths.
- Whenever you eat or drink something, take a minute and breathe. Look at your food and realize that the food was connected to something that nourished its growth. Can you see the sunlight, the rain, the earth, the farmer, the trucker in your food? Pay attention as you eat, consciously consuming this food for your physical health. Bring awareness to seeing your food, smelling your food, tasting your food, chewing your food, and swallowing your food.
- Notice your body while you walk or stand. Take a moment to notice your posture. Pay attention to the contact of the ground under your feet. Feel the air on your face, arms, and legs as you walk. Are you rushing?
- Bring awareness to listening and talking. Can you listen without agreeing or disagreeing, liking or disliking, or planning what you will say when it is your turn? When talking, can you just say what you need to say without overstating or understating? Can you notice how your mind and body feel?
- Whenever you wait in a line, use this time to notice standing and breathing. Feel the contact of your feet on the floor and how your body feels. Bring attention to the rise and fall of your abdomen. Are you feeling impatient?
- Be aware of any points of tightness in your body throughout the day. See if you can breathe into them and, as you exhale, let go of excess tension. Is there tension stored anywhere in your body? For example, your neck, shoulders, stomach, jaw, or lower back? If possible, stretch or do yoga once a day.
- Focus attention on your daily activities such as brushing your teeth, washing up, brushing your hair, putting on your shoes, doing your job. Bring mindfulness to each activity.
- Before you go to sleep at night, take a few minutes and bring your attention to your breathing. Observe five mindful breaths.

Adapted from Madeline Klyne, Instructor, Stress Reduction Clinic, University of Massachusetts Medical Center (personal communication). Copyright Madeline Klyne. Adapted by permission.

PART III

Evaluation and Dissemination

CHAPTER 14

❈

Mindfulness-Based Cognitive Therapy on Trial

Mulla Nasrudin, the wise fool of many teaching stories in the Middle East, was throwing handfuls of crumbs around his house, when a bemused onlooker asked him what he was doing. "Keeping the tigers away," the Mulla replied. "But surely there are no tigers in these parts," the onlooker responded. The Mulla beamed knowingly: "That's right. Effective, isn't it?"

As the story indicates, we can never be sure that actions intended to prevent some unwanted event are effective simply because the event does not occur—it might never have happened anyway. So, having developed the MBCT program to prevent future relapse to depression, how were we to find out whether our program delivered the desired effects? It was clear that simply running groups of recovered depressed patients through the program and counting how many relapsed in the following year, for example, would not tell us much—if there were few relapses, perhaps that is exactly what would have happened anyway; if there were many relapses, there might still have been fewer than if patients had not been through the program.

As you might expect, we were not the first to face such questions. Fortunately, a sophisticated methodology has been developed to address these issues, both in the evaluation of psychological treatments and in the assessment of the usefulness of clinical interventions more generally. At the heart of this methodology lies a process as random as tossing a coin.

THE POWER OF RANDOMIZATION

The randomized controlled trial (RCT) as a way to evaluate the effectiveness of clinical interventions was one of the most important developments in clinical and community medicine in the 20th century. In an RCT comparing the effectiveness of two treatments, the particular treatment that any patient receives, A or B, will be decided by a toss of a coin (or equivalently, by a computer-generated random sequence)—tails, the patient gets treatment A; heads, the patient gets treatment B. Patients then receive the treatment to which they have been allocated (having agreed in advance to their treatment being decided in this way). All patients are then assessed to determine the state of their clinical condition, and a score reflecting how well they are or how much improvement they have made is recorded. The numbers that have improved with treatment A and treatment B are then evaluated. Knowing the kind of differences that might be expected by chance alone, it is then possible to say, with a known level of confidence, that A is better than B, B is better than A, or that the difference between A and B is not greater than would be expected by chance. The more patients that there are in such a study, the more confident we can be in knowing that a difference of any given size between A and B is not simply due to chance. Equally, the greater number of patients that are studied, the more confident we can be that we have not missed the possibility of small, but possibly important, differences between treatments that might be attributed to chance with smaller numbers of patients.

In medicine, in evaluating a new drug, the two treatments compared in an RCT are commonly the new drug and a placebo pill that looks and tastes the same as the new drug but lacks its chemically active ingredients. If the RCT shows that patients who took the new drug improved more than those who took the placebo, then we can have some confidence that the active chemical ingredients of the drug contributed to those effects. It is, of course, essential in such trials that the person assessing the extent to which patients have improved does not know what kind of treatment (A or B) any given patient has received. Otherwise, his or her assessments might be biased by beliefs, conscious or unconscious, about the effectiveness of the two treatments—this is obviously likely to be a problem if the assessor has a financial or personal investment in the effectiveness of one treatment, for example, if he or she has invested many years in its development. For such reasons, in RCTs, assessments have to be made by assessors blind to treatment condition; that is, strenuous efforts have to be made to prevent assessors knowing or discovering the kind of treatment patients have actually received.

RANDOMIZED CONTROLLED TRIALS AND MINDFULNESS-BASED COGNITIVE THERAPY

In the simple but powerful RCT method, we had a way to overcome Nasrudin's error, the false belief that an action is effective in preventing an unwanted outcome, simply because the outcome does not occur. By randomly allocating recovered depressed patients to receive either the MBCT program or some comparison condition, and following them up to see how many people relapsed in the two groups, we would discover whether or not our efforts had paid off in producing an effective program.

But what should the comparison condition be? By analogy, with the conventional RCT to assess the effectiveness of a new drug, we would have compared MBCT with a placebo condition to see whether it had specific effects over and above the nonspecific effects of simply being in treatment, receiving attention from a health care professional, and so on. However, the use of placebo conditions in psychological treatment research in general, and in the evaluation of treatments for depression in particular, is much less straightforward than in the conventional drug trial. The difficulty is that, in a psychological treatment, many interlinked components cannot be separated from each other as easily as the chemically inert components of a pill can be separated from the potentially specific active drug that may also be mixed with them.

For example, we might think that one, specifically active psychological component of MBCT is learning how to relate from a decentered perspective to the negative thoughts and feelings that seem so important in precipitating relapse. This skill can only be learned by extensive homework practice. If we wanted to compare active MBCT with a "placebo" version of MBCT that also included homework, but did not teach decentering, we would immediately face the issue of what that homework should teach. For patients to be as actively engaged with "placebo" homework as with MBCT, that homework would have to make as much sense to them in relation to a wider understanding of relapse, and its prevention, as does decentering in relation to the overall rationale for MBCT. It is actually very difficult to find a placebo homework that is not, on the one hand, so obviously trivial and irrelevant that patients would not engage or persist with it, but that, on the other hand, while appearing relevant, does not involve procedures that we already know are likely to have effects on depression.

In fact, the choice of an appropriate comparison condition in an RCT will often be determined by the state of knowledge in a particular field at a particular time. At the time that we planned our RCT of MBCT, there was no published evidence that any psychological intervention offered to patients after recovery from depression could reduce future rates of relapse. This made our choice of a comparison condition easier. Before we needed to start worrying about whether MBCT, if effective, was effective for the specific reasons we thought, the first and most important step was to see whether it could produce better outcomes than the treatments that patients would normally receive. So we settled on a design for an RCT in which patients would be randomly allocated either simply to continue with the treatment that they would normally receive, or, in addition, be offered participation in the MBCT program. Those that were randomly allocated to the group that did not get MBCT were promised that they would have the chance to attend MBCT classes after the last follow-up data had been collected from their own and their comparison group.

So having worked out our general strategy for evaluating MBCT, what did we actually do, and what did we find?

OUR CLINICAL TRIAL OF MBCT

The aim of our trial (reported in detail in Teasdale and associates[80]) was to answer the question: Does MBCT reduce rates of relapse and recurrence in patients who have recovered from major depression, compared to the treatment that such patients would normally receive? Our initial calculations suggested that if we were to have a reasonable chance of coming up with a definite answer to this question, one way or the other, we would have to study a lot of patients. Specifically, considerations of statistical power told us that, if MBCT could, in reality, reduce relapse rates from 50% to 28%, we needed to have at least 120 patients completing both treatments if we wanted to have even an 80% chance of being sure of showing that difference, if it existed, in our trial. Given the inevitability of a proportion of patients dropping out before completing treatment, we knew that we would actually need to include a larger number than that in our trial. The only way we were going to get such numbers was by each of us offering MBCT to suitable patients at each of our three workplaces—Toronto, North Wales, and Cambridge—and pooling the results.

What Did We Do?

In our three-center clinical trial to evaluate MBCT, we recruited 145 patients who had recovered from major depression, that is, patients who had previously experienced episodes of major depression but had been well for the last 3 months, with no more symptoms of depression than one might expect of anyone in the normal population. These patients were randomly assigned to one of two conditions. In the first condition (treatment-as-usual), patients continued with the treatment that they would normally receive, including seeking help, as they needed it, from other sources, such as their family doctor. In the second condition, patients took part in the eight sessions of the MBCT program. To enter the trial, patients had to have had at least two previous episodes of major depression (in fact, 77% had experienced three or more). All patients had previously been treated with antidepressant medication but had been off medication for at least 3 months before entering the trial.

Before describing our results, we need to say a little more about one aspect of clinical trial methodology. In clinical trials such as the one we conducted, it is conventional to categorize each patient on certain baseline variables that might be related to the primary clinical outcome of interest before randomly assigning him or her to one treatment or another. The reason for using this procedure, known as "stratification," is to make sure that patients in the two treatment groups have comparable personal characteristics that are known to be associated with good or poor outcomes, regardless of the treatment they may receive. We were aware that the scientific literature on depression had identified two such factors, and so we decided to stratify based on (1) how recently the last episode of depression had occurred, and (2) how many previous episodes of major depression patients had experienced (two vs. three or more).

What Did We Find?

The outcome that most interested us was whether patients experienced a relapse or recurrence of their depression in the 60 weeks after their baseline assessment. As is conventional, before conducting the main statistical analyses of such a trial, we first checked that the effects of the treatments being compared were the same in patients in the different groups (strata) that stratification creates. When we did this, we found that, compared to treatment as usual, MBCT was not as effective in patients with only two previous episodes as in patients with three or more previous episodes of depression; there was a statistically significant difference between these two groups in the extent to which MBCT reduced relapse compared to treatment as usual. In patients with three or more episodes (77% of the total sample), MBCT significantly reduced relapse compared to treatment as usual; in patients with only two episodes (23% of the total sample), there was no difference in relapse rates between patients receiving MBCT and treatment as usual. In other words, the beneficial effects of MBCT were shown only in the patients with more extensive histories of depression. We had not expected this result. We consider possible explanations for this interesting finding below. For now, let us focus on the patients with three or more episodes, the considerable majority in the sample we studied (see Figure 14.1).

Of these, patients who simply continued with the treatment that they would normally have received showed a 66% relapse rate over

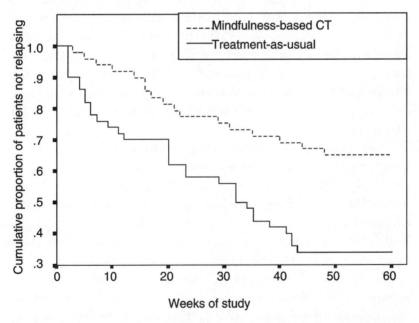

FIGURE 14.1. Survival curves comparing relapse/recurrence to DSM-III-R major depression for treatment as usual and mindfulness-based cognitive therapy, in patients with three or more previous episodes of major depression. From Teasdale et al.[80] Copyright 2000 by the American Psychological Association. Reprinted by permission.

the total 60-week study period, whereas those who received MBCT showed a relapse rate of 37%. The probability that we would get a difference this large by chance (if there were no real difference) was less than 1 in 200. Adding MBCT to the treatment that patients would normally receive had the effect of reducing risk of relapse almost by half. Furthermore, the greater use of antidepressants by patients in the MBCT group did not account for benefits of MBCT; the proportion of patients using antidepressants at any time during the study period was actually less in MBCT than in treatment-as-usual patients.

These findings were very heartening. In considering their implications, it is important to remember that MBCT was specifically designed for patients who had been depressed in the past but were relatively well at the time that they started the MBCT program. In particular, it is important to caution against interpreting our findings to support the use of MBCT with patients who are acutely depressed. At the moment, we have no evidence to suggest that MBCT would be useful with this group. Indeed, our best guess is that MBCT is unlikely to be effective in the treatment of acute depression, where factors such as difficulties in concentration and the intensity of negative thinking may make it very difficult for patients to develop the attentional skills central to the program.

The most important finding of our trial was that, in participants with three or more previous episodes of depression (who made up more than 75% of the patients we studied), MBCT almost halved relapse/recurrence rates over the follow-up period compared to treatment as usual. Because the patients were seen in groups, this benefit was much more cost-efficient than if patients had been seen individually, in the one-on-one format of conventional cognitive therapy for depression. Indeed, MBCT was able to help up to 12 patients in approximately the same time as it often takes to treat just one patient in conventional individual cognitive therapy for depression. So, it appeared that, for patients with three or more previous episodes of depression, we had achieved our aim of developing a new, cost-efficient way to reduce risk of relapse/recurrence of depression. But why was MBCT not helping patients with only two previous episodes of depression?

Why Did Mindfulness-Based Cognitive Therapy Not Help Patients with Only Two Previous Episodes of Depression?

We had not expected the benefits of MBCT to be restricted to patients with three or more previous episodes, not patients with only two previous episodes. We were able to come up with some plausible explanations for these findings (which we offer below), but we have to admit that, for now, these ideas are just that—unverified hunches that await further demonstrations and explorations of the pattern of results that we observed.

In patients in the treatment-as-usual group, risk of relapse and recurrence over the study period increased in a significant straight-line relationship with the number of previous episodes of depression they had experienced: The relapse/recurrence rate in patients with two episodes was 31%; in patients with three episodes, 56%; in patients with four or more episodes, 72%. In the group receiving MBCT, 37% of patients with more than two episodes relapsed, with no significant relationship between number of previous episodes and risk of relapse/recurrence: It seemed that the effect of MBCT was to eliminate the increased risk of relapse in patients with three or more previous episodes of depression.

The finding that MBCT prevented relapse/recurrence in patients with a history of three or more episodes of depression, but not in patients with only two previous episodes, is of particular interest with respect to the theoretical background to MBCT.[54,57] As we described in Chapter 2, the MBCT program was specifically designed to reduce the extent to which patterns of depressive thinking reactivated by sad moods could feed the factors responsible for relapse/recurrence. Such sadness-linked thinking, we assumed, resulted from repeated associations between the depressed state and characteristic negative thinking patterns within each depressive episode. Perhaps the strengthening of these associations with repeated episodes contributes to making relapse increasingly autonomous or automatic, so that it took less and less to actually trigger the return of symptoms. This view is supported by Post's observation that environmental stress appears to play a progressively less important role in bringing on relapse/recurrence with increasing number of episodes experienced.[33,81]

Such findings suggest the possibility that, in our trial of MBCT, (1) the greater risk of relapse in patients with three or more past episodes was to a large extent due to autonomous relapse processes involving reactivation of depressive thinking patterns by sad moods, and (2) the preventive effects of MBCT arose, specifically, from disruption of those processes at times of potential relapse/recurrence. Consistent with this analysis, MBCT appeared to have no prophylactic effects in patients with only two previous episodes of depression, and the rate to which relapse/recurrence was reduced by MBCT in those with three or more episodes (37%) was similar to the rate of relapse/recurrence in patients with only two previous episodes receiving treatment as usual (31%). Within this analysis, it is possible that relapse in patients with only two previous episodes of depression may have been substantially related to the occurrence of major life events, such as breakdowns in relationships, rather than the reactivation of more autonomous, relapse-related processes. Because the MBCT program placed very little emphasis on teaching problem-solving skills related to avoiding or coping with the effects of major interpersonal life events, its relative lack of effectiveness in patients with only two previous episodes of depression might not be unexpected.

Although this explanation seems likely, it is important that we remain cautious. An alternative explanation for both the Post effect and our result is that there are different types of depression. Some types of depression may be more closely associated with reaction to life events (and correspond to patients with only two previous episodes of depression in our trial). Other types of depression may be brought about not so much by unpleasant events but by prolonged rumination (and correspond to patients with three or more previous episodes of depression in our trial). If MBCT is more suitable for those whose depression is brought about by rumination, then this has at least two implications. First, one might find that the risk of relapse in this "ruminative" group can be reduced even lower than the 31% found in those with only two previous episodes, the "event reactive" group. Second, we need to find alternative methods to help members of this latter group, who have severe reactions to unpleasant life events.

OUR TRIAL IN PERSPECTIVE

It is important to be clear about what we can and cannot conclude from the results of our trial of MBCT. We can conclude, with some confidence, that in patients who have previously experienced three or more previous episodes of major depression, the MBCT program can produce useful reductions in risk of relapse/recurrence compared to the treatment such patients would usually receive in the course of normal service delivery. This is the first, and most important, question that we wanted to answer in relation to the effectiveness of MBCT. We cannot conclude that these reductions were specifically the result of the mindfulness training in the MBCT program. As we pointed out earlier, the design of our trial does not allow us to say that MBCT produced better prevention of future depression than might have been produced by alternative procedures. We cannot be sure how many of our effects came from the support that patients gave to each other, the attention of a kindly health professional, and so on. We have a very strong impression that the benefits of MBCT did not come from such nonspecific therapeutic factors alone, but, at the moment, we cannot support that impression by empirical evidence. That is the task for future trials, with different designs or methods of analysis.

To our knowledge, the results of our trial provide the first demonstration that a group-based psychological intervention, initially administered to patients in the recovered state, can significantly reduce risk of future relapse/recurrence in patients with recurrent major depression. As we mentioned earlier, at the time that we planned our trial, there was actually no published evidence that any psychological intervention, initially administered in the recovered state, could affect the future course of major depression. Since then, Giovanni Fava and his colleagues[82] in Italy have published evidence on the efficacy of a form of individual cognitive therapy for depression they developed that focuses on enhancing well-being rather than targeting negative aspects of experience. It is administered to recovered patients as their antidepressant medication is gradually withdrawn. Their results show that it can also substantially reduce future risk of relapse/recurrence. Such evidence strengthens further our confidence that our initial strategic decision way back at the beginning of our deliberations, to allow pharmacological treatment for the acute episode to take its course, with the later introduction of psychological interventions designed to prevent relapse, has much to commend it.

To our knowledge, ours was also the first multicenter randomized clinical trial evaluating a mindfulness-based clinical intervention. From the 1960s onward, there have been numerous studies demonstrating benefits of meditation-related procedures.[83] However, these investigations usually studied forms of meditation that emphasized concentration rather than mindfulness. Herbert Benson's[84] early work, for example, presented evidence that meditation is a useful clinical technique for stress-related conditions such as heart disease. His idea was that teaching individuals to maintain a narrowly focused concentration on a single stimulus could induce a state of deep relaxation and reduce their reactivity to stress. Interest in these approaches declined somewhat when studies began to report relatively little difference between forms of relaxation training that included meditation-like components and those that did not.

Interest in clinical applications of mindfulness meditation has been more recent (at least in the West), and has been largely fueled by the pioneering work of Jon Kabat-Zinn and his colleagues at the UMass Medical Center. As people in the West became more familiar with the variety of Buddhist systems of meditation, it became clear that these systems often differed in important ways from the types of concentrative practices that helped increase access to a "relaxation response." These approaches that emphasize insight meditation are what have more generally been called mindfulness. As we have seen in this book, in mindfulness practice, the focus of a person's attention is opened to admit whatever enters experience, while at the same time, a stance of kindly curiosity allows the person to investigate whatever appears, without falling prey to automatic judgments or reactivity. Support for the effectiveness of mindfulness-based clinical care in disorders such as chronic pain, generalized anxiety, and panic has come largely from uncontrolled evaluations rather than randomized clinical trials. It is very pleasing that the positive results obtained in these studies can now also be demonstrated in randomized controlled trials such as our own.

CHAPTER 15

⚏

Going Further

FURTHER READING, WEBSITES, AND ADDRESSES

Perhaps the possibility of integrating mindfulness training with aspects of cognitive therapy as a way to reduce suffering and promote well-being has sparked your interest to the point that you wish to explore this possibility further. Here, we offer some suggestions to guide your further exploration. We have focused primarily on mindfulness training and its clinical applications, rather than on cognitive therapy, because cognitive approaches to therapy are now very well established and often incorporated into the basic training of mental health care professionals, and training opportunities are widely available.

Turning to mindfulness, the best way to find out more is, undoubtedly, to have your own ongoing practice. Our own experience has amply confirmed the wisdom of the advice that we received when we first visited Jon Kabat-Zinn and his colleagues at the UMass Medical Center—"If you want to use mindfulness training with your patients, first, do it yourself." Below, we outline how to get started, if you, too, decide to follow this advice. However, it is quite likely that you would like to find out a bit more before taking this step. If so, there are excellent sources of further information available.

The video of Bill Moyers's documentary *Healing from Within,* describing the MBSR Program at the UMass Medical Center, gives a very direct, accessible, and interesting view of what actually happens in that program (we use it with our own patients in Sessions 4 and 5). As well as showing what goes on within sessions, case histories and interviews with Jon Kabat-Zinn present the thinking behind the program. This video is available from Ambrose Video Publishing, 28 West 44th Street, Suite 2100, New York, NY 10036; telephone: 800-526-4663; fax: 212-768-9282; website: www.ambrosevideo.com.

Jon Kabat-Zinn's own book *Full Catastrophe Living*[64] describes the UMass MBSR program in a very accessible and engaging way. It is an excellent introduction to clinical applications of mindfulness training for instructors and patients alike, and is essential reading for anyone wishing to explore this approach further. Again, this book is an important resource that we use in the MBCT program.

Jon Kabat-Zinn has also written *Wherever You Go, There You Are*[63] (published in the United Kingdom as *Mindfulness Meditation for Everyday Life*). This wonderful book conveys beautifully the spirit of bringing mindfulness to everyday experience, together with suggestions for practice. Another excellent source for a more detailed description of insight meditation, the tradition from which clinical applications of mindfulness are most directly derived, is *Seeking the Heart of Wisdom: The Path of Insight Meditation* by Joseph Goldstein and Jack Kornfeld.[85]

And if you decide you would actually like to taste directly the practice of mindfulness training? The best way is to be taught face-to-face by an experienced meditation teacher (see later details of how to find one). However, you might like, first, to "do it yourself" using audiotapes of guided meditation instructions. Again, the material that is actually used in the MBCT program can be used here, providing, at once, both an excellent introduction to your own meditation practice and a direct sampling of the exercises used by patients in the program. The tapes come in two series, both recorded by Jon Kabat-Zinn. Series 1 consists of two 45-minute tapes (which are also used on the UMass MBSR program) that narrate a guided body scan, a guided meditation on the breath, body, sounds, thoughts, and choiceless awareness, together with two different sessions of guided mindful hatha yoga. Series 2 consists of five tapes (each from 10- to 30-minutes long) specifically designed for those with a more general (rather than clinical) interest in learning mindfulness meditation. Both series can be ordered from Stress Reduction Tapes, P.O. Box 547, Lexington, MA 02420; website: www.stressreductiontapes.com.

If you would like to take the "do-it-yourself" option even more seriously, an excellent, comprehensive, distance learning package, "Introduction to Insight Meditation," has been prepared by two of the most respected Western meditation teachers in this tradition, Sharon Salzberg and Joseph Goldstein. This 12-month course includes 12 audiocassettes (each with a talk on one side and a guided meditation on the other), a workbook, and personal guidance (by e-mail, mail, or cassette correspondence) from an experienced meditation instructor. This course is available from Sounds True, P.O. Box 8010, Department V6, Boulder, CO 80306-8010.

Ideally, one learns meditation from personal contact with an experienced meditation teacher. There are many different forms of meditation. Therefore, from the perspective of preparing oneself as a potential instructor of MBCT, it is important to choose a tradition and teacher that are compatible in spirit and form with the MBCT program. In practice, this likely means exploring the teachings offered by centers related to the westernized insight meditation tradition. Information about these centers can be obtained from the following: in North America: Insight Meditation Society, 1230 Pleasant Street, Barre, MA 01005, or Spirit Rock, P.O. Box 909, Woodacre, CA 94973; in Europe: Gaia House, West Ogwell, Newton Abbot, Devon, TQ12 6EN, England. Further information on each of these centers is available directly or via links from the following website: www.dharma.org.

What about learning how to apply mindfulness training clinically? At the time of this writing, there are no systematic training courses for instructors on how to deliver the MBCT program (we hope this situation will change). There are, however, a variety of training opportunities for instructors in MBSR. MBCT and MBSR share many features in common. Consequently, the professional training available for MBSR provides an excellent preparation for offering MBCT to clients. Further details of these MBSR training opportunities are available from Director of Professional Training, Center for Mindfulness in Medicine, Health Care, and Society, University of Massachusetts Medical School, Worcester, MA 01655. Instruction from experienced MBSR or MBCT practitioners is undoubtedly the best way to learn how to use these approaches effectively. Recognizing that this may not always be possible, a variety of creative alternative solutions to acquiring the necessary skills are also worth exploring. To our knowledge, the strategy of a group of interested professionals getting together to take themselves through the MBSR or MBCT program, using the available audiotapes, videos, and written materials, has been explored in a number of settings and can provide an effective launchpad for the development of skills in program delivery. This exercise can provoke enough interest and enthusiasm that group members may then wish to repeat the experience to nurture further their developing skills. Most usefully, this approach would subsequently include continuing peer supervision, and, as soon as possible, feedback from experienced instructors and participation in formal training programs as they become available. In common with all forms of professional training in mindfulness-based clinical applications, such do-it-yourself approaches are likely to depend crucially on participants having their own ongoing practice of mindfulness (insight) meditation—again, such personal practice is of enormous benefit if participants are able to share experiences with a peer support group of fellow practitioners, whether or not group members are also interested in clinical applications of mindfulness training.

Epilogue

As we near the end of the book, it is time to reflect on how things have gone since those early days when we first came together. Our aim was to find how we might best help prevent relapse for patients who had been depressed in the past and remained vulnerable to future episodes of depression. Looking back, the process we have been through in developing this approach has been a learning experience that has changed the way we, as research scientists, think about things. The process of discovery inherent in this approach has also affected many of our clinical colleagues who, like us, have been intrigued by the possibility of using mindfulness approaches in health care. And our patients, too, in what started as an attempt to get rid of the burden of depression, have experienced something that has increased their well-being in many unexpected areas of their lives. A commonality of experience crosses the usual boundaries between researchers, clinicians, and patients. Each has made discoveries from which he or she learned. It is interesting to speculate on how such convergence emerges.

In whatever role we find ourselves, the process of change starts with a general, often difficult to articulate feeling that not everything is as it should be; things could be better than they are. From such a feeling may arise a commitment to find a better way of handling things: We start out on a path to discover a better way. This project has, so to speak, been like a meeting of several such paths. On the first path was a group of mindfulness teachers interested in finding useful clinical applications of their work and encouraging scientific exploration of specific applications and adaptations. On the second path were some clinical researchers, dissatisfied with existing approaches for dealing with relapse in depression. On the third path were some clinicians looking for an approach that would increase well-being in their patients rather than merely deal with pathology. On the fourth path were people who, depressed many times in the past, had come to the conclusion that there must be a better way to handle their lives. At the outset of the project, these people did not know that others had begun a journey from another starting point, nor that they were to meet at this particular crossroad. But meet they did, and this book has been an attempt to say what happened as the result of the meeting.

The new possibilities we have explored appear to have taken us, in many ways, a long way away from our original home territory of cognitive therapy. We incorporated elements that explore mindfulness of the breath, of the body, of sounds, of emotional expression as it is happening, as well as thoughts, the more usual domain of cognitive work. We wanted participants to sample how each of these might be used in daily life to learn to pay attention in a different way: on purpose, in the present moment, and nonjudgmentally; to pay attention to what was going on in mind and body in a way that put analysis aside; to let whatever is here just be here, noticing how it changes and the way its hold gets stronger or weaker. By patient and persistent practice, we hoped that participants might explore how it is possible to relate differently to themselves and their difficulties.

Moving out of home territory is never easy, especially for clinicians who have found a way that seems comfortable for themselves and their patients.

Some years ago, in the early days of cognitive therapy, a senior clinician telephoned a young cognitive therapist. "Sorry to miss your training workshop last week," he said. "Call round to my office sometime and tell me about this cognitive therapy." Obediently, his young colleague made an appointment for 2 o'clock the next day.

The older man sat behind his large desk and listened while the young cognitive therapist explained principles and practices. After 5 minutes, he interrupted. "Ah, so that's what it is. I'm so glad to hear that I already do cognitive therapy. I often find my patients' thinking is distorted and I tell them so. Thank you very much for your time. Could you leave me some of those diaries and record forms on your way out?"

Years later, the young cognitive therapist had become more senior. He had written books about and given workshops about cognitive therapy all over the world. One day, someone mentioned that mindfulness meditation might be useful in helping those who are vulnerable to depression. "So tell me about it," he said. His informant did so. "It seems like just relaxation to me," he said. "And the bits that aren't relaxation seem to me to be cognitive therapy—and I already do that."

Remaining open to new possibilities as a clinician is difficult. Few people want to be seen as butterflies, flitting from one therapy to another, with the enthusiasm of the new convert, only to reject it a few months later when they hear the price of getting accredited! Yet if we believe that our aim should be to improve the effectiveness of treatments to bring about the peace, freedom, and well-being that people seek (and we still do not know a better motive for clinical research), then openness to new approaches is not an enemy. Rather, it is a vital challenge to keep searching for new ways to help more people. People who seek help from us deserve no less.

Those who come asking us for help have often tried so many times to get on top of their problems that they are beginning to wonder whether anything can help. They have often interpreted their previous difficulties as a basic failure in themselves. Often, they have long given up thinking well of themselves, thinking of themselves as worthy of love. The book refers many times to the fact that we wished to cultivate in each participant an attitude of kindness to him- or herself. But what a curious place to start: to illustrate the need to wake up to each moment by asking people to eat a raisin mindfully! Yet we learned never to underestimate the power of small actions, for each moment might contain the seed of something much greater than itself. As it turns out, the wisdom that helps us to deal with tragedies and disappointments is the same wisdom that sees, in the ordinary and everyday things of life, how things change from one moment to the next, often in surprising ways. We have finished the story of the journey we began in the first chapter of this book. Our hope is that we have conveyed enough of the spirit of this approach to allow you also to feel that it may someday also be a journey worth taking.

References

1. Teasdale JD, Barnard P. *Affect, cognition and change*. Hove, UK: Erlbaum, 1993.
2. Lepine JP, Gastpar M, Mendlewicz J, Tylee A. Depression in the community: The first pan-European study DEPRES. *International Clinical Psychopharmacology* 1997; *12*:19–29.
3. Parikh SV, Wasylenki D, Goering P, Wong J. Mood disorders: Rural/urban differences in prevalence, health care utilization and disability in Ontario. *Journal of Affective Disorders* 1996; *38*:57–65.
4. Weissman MM, Bruce LM, Leaf PJ. Affective disorders. In Robins LN, Regier DA, eds. *Psychiatric disorders in America: The Epidemiologic Catchment Area study*. New York: Free Press, 1990:53–80.
5. Kessler RC, McGonagle KA, Zhao S, et al. Lifetime and twelve-month prevalence of DSM-III-R psychiatric disorders in the United States: Results from the National Comorbidity Study. *Archives of General Psychiatry* 1994; *51*:8–19.
6. Consensus Development Panel. NIMH/NIH consensus development conference statement: Mood disorders—Pharmacologic prevention of recurrence. *American Journal of Psychiatry* 1985; *142*:469–476.
7. Keller MB, Lavori PW, Mueller TI, Coryell W, Hirschfeld RMA, Shea MT. Time to recovery, chronicity and levels of psychotherapy in major depression. *Archives of General Psychiatry* 1992; *49*:809–816.
8. Sargeant JK, Bruce ML, Florio LP, Weissman MM. Factors associated with 1-year outcome for major depression in the community. *Archives of General Psychiatry* 1990; *47*:519–526.

9. Boyd JH, Burke JD, Gruneberg E, et al. Exclusion criteria of DSM-III: A study of co-occurrence of hierarchy-free syndromes. *Archives of General Psychiatry* 1984; *41*:983–959.

10. Murray CL, Lopez AD. *The global burden of disease: A comprehensive assessment of mortality and disability from disease, injuries and risk factors in 1990 and projected to 2020.* Boston: Harvard University Press, 1998.

11. Wells KB, Sturm R, Sherbourne CD, Meredith LS. *Caring for depression.* Boston: Harvard University Press, 1996.

12. Broadhead WE, Blazer DG, George LK, Tse CK. Depression, disability days and days lost from work in a prospective epidemiological survey. *Journal of the American Medical Association* 1990; *264*:2524–2528.

13. Stansfeld SA, Fuhrer R, Head J, Ferrie J, Shipley M. Work and psychiatric disorder in the Whitehall II study. *Journal of Psychosomatic Research* 1997; *43*:73–81.

14. Nathan KI, Musselman DL, Schatzberg AF, Nemeroff CB. Biology of mood disorders. In Nemeroff CB, ed. *The American Psychiatric Press textbook of psychopharmacology.* Washington, DC: American Psychiatric Press, 1995:439–478.

15. Healy D. *The antidepressant era.* Cambridge, MA: Harvard University Press, 1997.

16. Lewinsohn PM, Antonuccio DO, Steinmetz JL, Teri L. *The Coping with Depression course: A psychoeducational intervention for unipolar depression.* Eugene, OR: Castalia Press, 1984.

17. Becker RE, Heimberg RG, Bellack AS. *Social skills training treatment for depression.* Elmsford, NY: Pergamon Press, 1987.

18. Beck AT, Rush AJ, Shaw BF, Emery G. *Cognitive therapy of depression.* New York: Guilford Press, 1979.

19. Klerman GL, Weissman MM, Rounsaville BJ, Chevron E. *Interpersonal psychotherapy of depression.* New York: Basic Books, 1984.

20. Rehm LP. A self-control model of depression. *Behavior Therapy* 1977; *8*:787–804.

21. Williams JMG. *The psychological treatment of depression.* London: Routledge, 1992.

22. Keller MB, Lavori PW, Lewis CE, Klerman GL. Predictors of relapse in major depressive disorder. *Journal of the American Medical Association* 1983; *250*:3299–3304.

23. Paykel ES, Ramana R, Cooper Z, Hayhurst H, Kerr J, Barocka A. Residual symptoms after partial remission: An important outcome in depression. *Psychological Medicine* 1995; *25*:1171–1180.

24. Judd LL. The clinical course of unipolar major depressive disorders. *Archives of General Psychiatry* 1997; *54*: 989–991.

25. Coryell W, Endicott J, Keller MB. Outcome of patients with chronic affective disorder: A five year follow up. *American Journal of Psychiatry* 1990; *147*:1627–1633.

26. American Psychiatric Association. *Diagnostic and statistical manual of mental disorders—Text revision*. Washington, DC: American Psychiatric Press, 2000.

27. Thase ME, Kupfer DJ, Buysse DJ, et al. Electroencephalographic sleep profiles in single-episode and recurrent unipolar forms of depression: 1. Comparison during acute depressive states. *Biological Psychiatry* 1995; *1*:72–80.

28. Glen AI, Johnson AL, Shepherd M. Continuation therapy with lithium and amitriptyline in unipolar depressive illness: A randomized, double blind, controlled trial. *Psychological Medicine* 1984; *14*:37–50.

29. Frank E, Prien RF, Jarrett RB, et al. Conceptualization and rationale for consensus definitions of terms in major depressive disorder. *Archives of General Psychiatry* 1991; *48*:851–855.

30. American Psychiatric Association. Practice guidelines for the treatment of patients with major depressive disorder (revision). *American Journal of Psychiatry* 2000; *157*:1–45.

31. Hollon SD, Shelton RC, Loosen PT. Cognitive therapy and pharmacotherapy for depression. *Journal of Consulting and Clinical Psychology* 1991; *59*:88–99.

32. Prien RF, Kupfer DJ, Mansky PA, et al. Drug therapy in the prevention of recurrences in unipolar and bipolar affective disorders: Report of the NIMH Collaborative Study Group comparing lithium carbonate, imipramine and a lithium carbonate–imipramine combination. *Archives of General Psychiatry* 1984; *41*:1096–1104.

33. Post RM. Transduction of psychosocial stress into the neurobiology of recurrent affective disorder. *American Journal of Psychiatry* 1992; *149*: 999–1010.

34. Lin EH, Von Korff M, Katon W, Bush T, Simon GE, Walker E, Robinson P. The role of the primary care physician in patients' adherence to antidepressant therapy. *Medical Care* 1995; *33*:67–74.

35. Basco MR, Rush AJ. Compliance with pharmacology in mood disorders. *Psychiatric Annals* 1995; *25*:269–275.

36. Reuters/Health. Few patients satisfied with antidepressants, 1999. Available: www.reuters.com.

37. Frank E, Kupfer DJ, Perel JM, et al. Three year outcomes for mainte-
    nance therapies in recurrent depression. *Archives of General Psychiatry*
    1990; *47*:1093–1099.

38. Frank E, Kupfer DJ, Wagner EF, McEachran AB, Cornes C. Efficacy of
    interpersonal psychotherapy as a maintenance treatment of recurrent
    depression: Contributing factors. *Archives of General Psychiatry* 1991;
    48:1053–1059.

39. Jarrett RB, Basco MR, Risser R, et al. Is there a role for continuation
    phase cognitive therapy for depressed outpatients? *Journal of Con-
    sulting and Clinical Psychology* 1998; *66*:1036–1040.

40. Blackburn IM, Eunson KM, Bishop S. A two-year naturalistic follow-up
    of depressed patients treated with cognitive therapy, pharmacotherapy,
    and a combination of both. *Journal of Affective Disorders* 1986; *10*:67–75.

41. Evans MD, Hollon SD, DeRubeis J, et al. Differential relapse following
    cognitive therapy and pharmacotherapy for depression. *Archives of
    General Psychiatry* 1992; *49*:802–808.

42. Shea MT, Elkin I, Imber S, et al. Course of depressive symptoms over fol-
    low up: Findings from the NIMH treatment of depression collaborative
    research program. *Archives of General Psychiatry* 1992; *49*:782–787.

43. Simons A, Murphy G, Levine J, Wetzel R. Cognitive therapy and
    pharmacotherapy for depression: Sustained improvement over one year.
    Archives of General Psychiatry 1986; *43*:43–50.

44. Beck AT. *Cognitive therapy and the emotional disorders*. New York: In-
    ternational Universities Press, 1976.

45. Kovacs MB, Beck AT. Maladaptive cognitive structures in depression.
    American Journal of Psychiatry 1978; *135*:525–533.

46. Weissman M, Beck AT. *Development and validation of the Dysfunctional
    Attitude Scale*. Paper presented at the meeting of the Association for Ad-
    vancement of Behavior Therapy, Chicago, 1978.

47. Ingram RE, Miranda J, Segal ZV. *Cognitive vulnerability to depression*.
    New York: Guilford Press, 1998.

48. Teasdale JD. Negative thinking in depression: Cause, effect or recipro-
    cal relationship? *Advances in Behaviour Research and Therapy* 1983;
    5:3–25.

49. Teasdale JD. Cognitive vulnerability to persistent depression. *Cognition
    and Emotion* 1988; *2*:247–274.

50. Segal ZV, Ingram RE. Mood priming and construct activation in tests of
    cognitive vulnerability to unipolar depression. *Clinical Psychology Re-
    view* 1994; *14*:663–695.

51. Miranda J, Persons JB. Dysfunctional attitudes are mood state dependent. *Journal of Abnormal Psychology* 1988; 97:76–79.

52. Miranda J, Persons JB, Byers C. Endorsement of dysfunctional beliefs depends on current mood state. *Journal of Abnormal Psychology* 1990; 99:237–241.

53. Segal ZV, Gemar MC, Williams S. Differential cognitive response to a mood challenge following successful cognitive therapy or pharmacotherapy for unipolar depression. *Journal of Abnormal Psychology* 1999; *108*:3–10.

54. Segal ZV, Williams JMG, Teasdale JD, Gemar MC. A cognitive science perspective on kindling and episode sensitization in recurrent affective disorder. *Psychological Medicine* 1996; 26:371–380.

55. Nolen-Hoeksema S, Morrow J. A prospective study of depression and posttraumatic stress symptoms after a natural disaster: The 1989 Loma Prieta earthquake. *Journal of Personality and Social Psychology* 1991; *61*:115–121.

56. Lyubomirsky S, Nolen-Hoeksema S. Effects of self-focused rumination on negative thinking and interpersonal problem solving. *Journal of Personality and Social Psychology* 1995; 69:176–190.

57. Teasdale JD, Segal ZV, Williams JMG. How does cognitive therapy prevent relapse and why should attentional control (mindfulness) training help? *Behaviour Research and Therapy* 1995; *33*:225–239.

58. Barber JP, DeRubeis, R. On second thought: Where the action is in cognitive therapy. *Cognitive Therapy and Research* 1989; *13*:441–457.

59. Simons AD, Garfield S, Murphy G. The process of change in cognitive therapy and pharmacotherapy for depression. *Archives of General Psychiatry* 1984; *49*:45–51.

60. Ingram RE, Hollon SD. Cognitive therapy for depression from an information processing perspective. In Ingram RE, ed. *Information processing approaches to clinical psychology.* Orlando, FL: Academic Press, 1986:261–284.

61. Linehan MM, Armstrong HE, Suarez A, Allmon D, Heard H. Cognitive-behavioral treatment of chronically parasuicidal borderline patients. *Archives of General Psychiatry* 1991; *48*:1060–1064.

62. Linehan MM. *Cognitive-behavioral treatment of borderline personality disorder.* New York: Guilford Press, 1993.

63. Kabat-Zinn J. *Wherever you go, there you are: Mindfulness meditation in everyday life.* New York: Hyperion, 1994.

64. Kabat-Zinn J. *Full castastrophe living: Using the wisdom of your body*

and mind to face stress, pain, and illness. New York: Dell Publishing, 1990.

65. Kabat-Zinn J, Massion AO, Kristeller J, et al. Effectiveness of a meditation-based stress reduction program in the treatment of anxiety disorders. *American Journal of Psychiatry* 1992; *149*:936–943.

66. Kabat-Zinn J, Lipworth L, Burney R, Sellers W. Four-year follow-up of a meditation-based program for self-regulation of chronic pain: Treatment outcomes and compliance. *Clinical Journal of Pain* 1986; *2*:159–173.

67. Miller J, Fletcher K, Kabat-Zinn J. Three year follow up and clinical implications of a mindfulness-based stress reduction intervention in the treatment of anxiety disorders. *General Hospital Psychiatry* 1995; *17*:192–200.

68. McLean P, Hakstian A. Clinical depression: Relative efficacy of outpatient treatments. *Journal of Consulting and Clinical Psychology* 1979; *47*:818–836.

69. Watzlawick P, Fisch R, Weakland J. *Change: Priniciples of problem formation and problem resolution.* New York: Norton, 1974.

70. Wegner D. Ironic processes of mental control. *Psychological Review* 1994; *101*:34–52.

71. Rosenberg L. *Breath by breath.* Boston: Shambhala, 1998.

72. Roskos-Ewoldsen DE, Fazio RH. On the orienting value of attitudes: Attitude accessibility as a determinant of an object's attraction of visual attention. *Journal of Personality and Social Psychology* 1992; *63*:198–211.

73. Hollon SD, Kendall P. Cognitive self-statements in depression: Development of an Automatic Thoughts Questionnaire. *Cognitive Therapy and Research* 1980; *4*:383–395.

74. Goldstein J. *Insight meditation.* Boston: Shambhala, 1994.

75. Oliver M. *Dream work.* Boston: Grove/Atlantic, 1986.

76. Santorelli S. *Heal thyself: Lessons on mindfulness in medicine.* New York: Bell Tower, 1999.

77. Barks C, Moyne J. *The essential Rumi.* San Francisco: Harper, 1997.

78. Fennell M. Depression. In Hawton K, Salkovskis P, Kirk J, Clark D, eds. *Cognitive behaviour therapy for psychiatric problems.* Oxford, UK: Oxford University Press, 1989:169–234.

79. Oliver M. *House of light.* Boston: Beacon Press, 1990.

80. Teasdale JD, Segal ZV, Williams JMG, Ridgeway V, Soulsby J, Lau M. Prevention of relapse/recurrence in major depression by mindfulness-based cognitive therapy. *Journal of Consulting and Clinical Psychology* 2000; *68*:615–623.

81. Kendler KS, Thornton LM, Gardner CO. Stressful life events and previous episodes in the etiology of major depression in women: An evaluation of the "kindling" hypothesis. *American Journal of Psychiatry* 2000; *157*:1243–1251.

82. Fava G, Grandi S, Zielezny M, Rafanelli C, Canestrari R. Four-year outcome for cognitive behavioural treatment of residual symptoms in primary major depressive disorder. *American Journal of Psychiatry* 1996; *153*:945–947.

83. Loizzo J. Meditation and psychotherapy. In Muskin P, ed. *Review of psychiatry. Vol. 19*. Washington, DC: American Psychiatric Association Press, 2000:147–197.

84. Benson H. Systematic hypertension and the relaxation response. *New England Journal of Medicine* 1977; 296:1152–1156.

85. Goldstein J, Kornfeld J. *Seeking the heart of wisdom: The path of insight meditation*. Boston: Shambhala, 1987.

Index